Managing Your Emotional Health Using Traditional Chinese Medicine

How Herbs, Natural Foods, and Acupressure
Can Regulate and Harmonize Your Mind and Body

Zhang Yifang

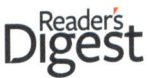

The Reader's Digest Association, Inc.
Pleasantville, New York / Montreal / Sydney

Copyright © 2010 Shanghai Press & Publishing Development Company
The Reader's Digest Association, Inc., is the authorized publisher of the English-language edition outside China.

All rights reserved. Unauthorized reproduction, in any manner, is prohibited.

Reader's Digest is a registered trademark of The Reader's Digest Association, Inc.

FOR SHANGHAI PRESS & PUBLISHING DEVELOPMENT COMPANY
President and Publisher: Wang Youbu
Editorial Director: Wu Ying
Editors: Ye Jiasheng, Kirstin Mattson

Text: Zhang Yifang
Photographs: Roger Yan, Zhang Yifang, Roy Upton, Alfred Kump, Yao Yingzhi, Herbasinica, Quanjing, istockphoto.com

Interior Designers: Yuan Yinchang, Li Jing, Hu Bin

ISBN 978-1-60652-162-5
Library of Congress Cataloging-in-Publication Data is available upon request.

FOR READER'S DIGEST
Executive Editor, Trade Publishing: Dolores York
Cover Design: George Mckeon

THE READER'S DIGEST ASSOCIATION, INC.
President and Chief Executive Officer: Mary Berner
President of Asia Pacific: Andrea Martin
President and Publisher, U.S. Trade Publishing: Harold Clarke

Printed in China by Shenzhen Donnelley Printing Co. Ltd.

1 3 5 7 9 10 8 6 4 2

To my husband Jianwei

Contents

Acknowledgments 7

Introduction 9

Chapter 1 Managing Emotions according to Constitution and Temperament 16

Chapter 2 Managing Emotions through the Five Elements: the Heart System 32

Chapter 3 Managing Emotions through Yin-Yang Theory: the Lung System 46

Chapter 4 Managing the Complex Emotional Cycle: the Liver System 60

Chapter 5 Managing Emotions throughout Your Life Cycle: the Kidney System 76

Chapter 6 Managing Emotions according to Gender: the Digestive System (Spleen) 90

Chapter 7 Managing Emotions according to the Seasons 108

Appendices Yin-Yang Theory 123
Five Elements Theory 126
Five Systems of the Body 130
Brief Patient Diagnosis 131
Different Constitutions and Temperaments 132
Helpful Acupressure Points 134
Chinese Food and Herbs 136
Bibliography 150

Acknowledgments

Any piece of work is always a collaboration, so I would like to thank the people who helped contribute to the compilation of this book. First, I would like to thank my grandfather who influenced me through his knowledge and successful practice when I was a little girl. Secondly, I want to thank my father for his guidance and encouragement, and for sharing his life experiences learning and working in TCM for decades in China, and also my mother for giving me confidence and support. Thirdly, I want to thank my husband for encouraging me to learn English in a quick and practical way for use in my TCM career. He devoted a lot of time to inspiring me how to go about writing this book. My daughter was also a great help in this endeavor, spending hours on the internet and with my medical books to help me research findings.

Many thanks, too, to Amena Lee Schlaikjer for contributing her thoughts and knowledge of Eastern and Western cultures. We spent a good time together on weekend mornings (in addition to late evenings on her own to make this process quicker and more fluid) writing this book through dictation.

I would like to thank Roger Yan, a friend and artist, who created the beautiful drawings for this book to bring my words to life and add a little more art to science. A portion of the pictures of herbs and plants appear thanks to Roy Upton, the Executive Director of American Herbal Pharmacopoeia. The Appendices and accumulation of part of the theory was done by my wonderful assistant, Anna Zhao, who put in many hours to help me—I thank her for this effort.

Introduction

Why have I decided to sum up 25 years of research and clinical practice, three generations of experience and 5000 years of Chinese philosophy and medicine in this book?

Firstly, I write this in response to the continuous unbalanced way of living we have created in the modern world, and to bring back an age-old, proven science that provides a natural solution to remedy this instability.

Finding a way to maintain a positive spirit and a healthy lifestyle has become an increasingly important focus these days. Traditional Chinese Medicine (TCM), which has been relied upon by millions of people over the generations, provides simple yet effective ways to achieve optimal health.

TCM focuses on the organic whole of the person, physiologically and psychologically, to bring the individual in balance with nature and society. It emphasizes natural remedies—food and herbs—as well as adjusting the mind, before treating with medicine, because the latter is often accompanied by side effects. In this way, without unnatural chemicals, you can maintain an optimistic outlook, dissolve negative moods and unhealthy habits, and keep your mind and body in balance.

In particular, I want to address the natural remedial management of our emotions, a subject that has not received much attention in English-language books. Building on my father's many years as a successful doctor in this arena, I have devoted my personal attention to this area of study, for which there is increasing demand.

TCM in China has a long history of managing emotional changes that are not just mental but also based on the physical body and its natural cycles. TCM manages emotions naturally, treating the body rather than just focusing on the mind, as they are both intrinsically linked. Many conditions that Western medicine labels as "mental diseases" or "emotional diseases" are instead recognized by TCM as imbalances in the body that provoke a resulting surge of emotion, or disturbed internal system of qi*, the energy or life-process that flows in and around all of us. Emotions can be handled by balancing qi throughout the body and its organs, providing a natural and holistic remedy.

The second reason I have written this book is to let people know that emotional changes are normal for everyone. We live in a busy world, and our emotions may change as our environment or body changes. Emotions are inevitable, abundant and part of a valuable life experience. No matter what kind of emotion you have, it influences everyone around you. If you want to achieve your career goals and maintain harmony with your family, friends and colleagues, you have to manage your emotions. Otherwise, life is less enjoyable—for example, if you are unable to relax with your family and friends, or become unable to do the things you like to do. So emotional management is a part of life management: It helps prevent moods that can make you feel overwhelmed, withdrawn or unbalanced, and allows for a more productive and fulfilling life.

People feel that worry, panic, fear, anxiety and depression are all symptoms to be avoided, and in some countries, are diagnosed as diseases with convenient one-pill remedies. However, these emotions are entirely natural—they have had a purpose from the beginning of time and throughout our evolution. They are therefore natural components of our life, and they have their advantages in our personal development. For example, some amounts of stress are good, and can cause physical and mental responses that actually make a person perform better in difficult circumstances.

This book will help you decide when you should see a doctor and when you can handle things by yourself. People have the misconception that happiness is the only emotion we are supposed to feel, and that any other emotion is solved with pills. Many emotions can be easily managed by increasing intake of specific herbs and being aware of your diet, starting exercise therapies outdoors with exposure to sunlight, and changing certain lifestyle habits. Quitting smoking, removing cold foods from your diet, and eating a healthy breakfast can actually have a profound impact on one's health. Sometimes, having contact with others, or just sharing emotions with friends is all it takes to improve your emotional well-being.

When one suffers stress from studying, working, worrying or poor habits, which frequently are the "norm" in the modern world, TCM will often have a direct and personalized answer. For instance, the simple act of missing breakfast due to rushing to work can actually offset one's entire flow of qi, and therefore emotional balance, for the day. While if breakfast is eaten late, the stress may only be short-lived, missing it entirely can ruin the whole day, and even become a new habit that is difficult to change. Over time, this will actually have lasting negative effects on one's constitution and temperament.

In order to manage stress, each person must focus attention on daily lifestyle habits and a thorough understanding of one's own constitution. There are seven different kinds of constitutions: cold, hot, weak, dry, damp, complicated and balanced. People usually fall within the parameters of these seven groups.

Mood starts with your physical body, and changing one's constitution starts with food. Then other remedies that affect mood, like listening to music, social interaction and massages, will help more. Environmental factors can affect mood but mostly they are just enhancers. The body is highly adaptable so the environment takes a long time to start having an effect. However, working to change one's internal constitution can bring improvements more effectively and efficiently. Starting with good food is a first step to change overall health for the better, but one must understand his or her own constitution in order to take the right steps to enhance one's life and find good, lasting health.

Thirdly, this is not a book that promises to provide an overarching look at TCM theory nor is it a complete resource on self-diagnosis or treatment. However, I hope it will serve as an important tool in managing your emotional health.

The following ten cases are only a small selection from years of practice and training in TCM emotional management. I wish I could share more, but I specifically chose ones that best exemplify the different management systems to cope with common imbalances in our lives. Each chapter concentrates on a segment of research. Starting with an old TCM proverb, the chapters then present case stories followed by simple analysis, and conclude with advice on the type of treatment or remedy that would help in general cases. Some food and lifestyle recommendations follow, but in general, it is always good to consult a TCM practitioner and Western doctor to fully understand your symptoms and general health before proceeding with a treatment program.

I would like to introduce some of TCM's most important

underlying concepts here to help you better understand the case stories, analysis and remedies presented in the following chapters. You may also turn to the Appendices for more information.

A cornerstone of TCM is yin-yang theory, an ancient philosophical concept stating that there are two fundamental principles or forces in the universe, ever opposing and supplementing each other. All things and phenomena in the natural world contain two opposite components, for example, heaven and earth, outside and inside, heat and cold, etc.

In TCM, yin and yang can be used to explain the body's composition, its physiological functions and pathology changes. TCM's clinical diagnosis seeks to determine if yin and yang are balanced. If imbalances are found, its treatments focus on restoring equilibrium through the use of foods, herbs and other methods. For example, a food that strengthens yin energy may be used against a disease caused by an excess of yang.

Another theory that forms an important component of TCM practice is Five Elements theory. According to this ancient theory, wood, fire, earth, metal and water are the five basic substances that constitute the material world. They each have their own unique properties and they also have specific relationships with one another: generation, restriction, subjugation and reverse restriction.

TCM has made a comprehensive study of all things in nature, including the human body, and attributed each to one of the Five Elements. For example, the heart, the emotion of joy and the season of summer are classified as "fire," while the lung, worry and autumn are considered "metal." TCM uses these classifications and relationships to guide the diagnosis and treatment of physical and psychological conditions. For example, in Five Elements theory, fire restricts metal, so a treatment may use joy (fire) to treat a case of sadness or over-worry (metal).

In TCM, diagnosis and treatment also rely on the concepts of constitution and temperament. An individual's constitution is based on the relative strength of yin-yang energies and different movements of qi and blood in the body. To understand your own constitution according to TCM, you can consult my website, www.acherbs.com, where you can take two short assessments. These will give you a personalized reference point in understanding how to achieve better health, as remedies (such as foods and herbs) are tailored to specific constitutions.

As you can see, the concepts behind Traditional Chinese Medicine differ greatly from Western medicine. TCM doctors rely on an entirely different diagnostic technique, *wang wen wen qie*, which means that to gauge the health of a patient, one incorporates looking, smelling, hearing, feeling and asking everything about the patient's life. They integrate psychological explanations and the state of their patient's physical body to understand the unbalanced qi flow, ultimately shedding a different light on how patients can better take control of their physical and emotional health.

However, modern practitioners integrate the wisdom of TCM with the fruit of modern research. They strive to use the best of both Chinese and Western medical approaches to help people maintain a balance of the body and mind, achieve harmony with the natural world and avoid deterioration into illness.

I do want to mention that all of China's top TCM universities have innovatively combined the modern adaptations of TCM with advances in Western medicine. They now teach a curriculum that is based up to 40% on Western medicine, so that the understanding of the body is more well-rounded. Perhaps this is an approach that Western medicine should also consider.

Traditional Chinese Medicine is a treasure accumulated over 5000 years and it deserves to be shared by the people on this planet. In this era of globalization, we are facing many issues, which cause emotional disturbances that require better solutions through a combination of traditional wisdom and modern knowledge. The business of emotional management through TCM is a business of humanity. I hope this book will not only inspire others to work on bettering their own health but also bring forth ideas and new research to better the lives of everyone.

In Chinese we say, *"qian li zhi xing shi yu zu xia,"* which means that if you have a great goal, you must start walking towards it today! This book's straightforward and practical approach will give you the tools you need to achieve a satisfying and balanced life. By making a few simple changes, you will find a rapid and noticeable improvement in your emotional well-being. So join us in exploring how to develop a proactive attitude toward treatment and prevention, and bring more enjoyment to your life!

Dr. Zhang Yifang

---

* I will use the accepted pinyin spelling, "qi" of the word often known as "chi" (in the Wade–Giles romanization system), "ki" (in Japanese), or "gi" (in Korean).

Chapter 1
Managing Emotions according to Constitution and Temperament

脏气有强弱，禀赋有阴阳。

——张介宾

Zang qi you qiang ruo, bing fu you yin yang.

The qi of the internal organs can be strong or weak; the congenital natural disposition of human beings is classified into yin or yang.

—Zhang Jiebin

The internal organs, energy, blood and functions of each person have different relative levels of strength. For instance, some people's hearts are stronger than other people's, and also, their hearts may be stronger than other organs in their own bodies. One person may have a higher tolerance for spicy food or alcohol than another; this person's body can handle the excess intake as opposed to others whose system may not be strong enough to cope. Therefore, people's constitutions can show cold or hot, dry or damp tendencies—having different reactions to different circumstances.

Case Story 1

Salesman David came to China to open his trading company and tried to sell American luxury brands that were less known in China. Although he was experienced in this business at home, he struggled in an unfamiliar environment and felt lonely and anxious. Theoretically, China is an enormous and exciting market, but landing business here is far from easy: a difficult language, lots of regulation and indirect communication, narrowed social networking and high financial pressures. David had to work long hours and attended a lot of business meetings and dinners in addition to often going on business trips. Even on the weekends, his mind was still busy with ideas and planning for the following week.

After half a year, David regularly felt tired, lacked motivation and enthusiasm, and lost his temper easily. In order to alleviate the pressure, David started to drink alcohol and smoke, but worried even more. One day when he was ready to attend a meeting, he suddenly started to experience palpitations, sweaty palms and a high-pitched sound in his ear along with lower back pain. He decided to rest that day and felt much better, except for the noise in his ear. Since then, whenever he has important business meetings, he can't sleep well, finding it difficult both to fall sleep and remain asleep, waking up early. How can he cope with this type of life and carry on with his business?

Case Story 2

Sarah, a housewife, was a very shy person. After her second childbirth, she wanted to quickly lose the pregnancy weight, and become a vegetarian. During that time, her mother's fight with cancer escalated. Sarah felt guilty and sad that she was unable to care for her, and that her mother's passing happened so quickly. Around the same time, a bomb exploded in a city that was far away from her town, but still induced an extreme fear of sudden catastrophes. From that point on, she refused to go on any airplanes, cars or trains, only living in her small town and doing errands by foot. Even sudden sounds like car honking or loud bells would cause her to shake and palpitate. She also lost a lot of weight during that time due to poor sleep accompanied by nightmares.

Analysis

The above cases illustrate instances of extreme phobia. In TCM, there are two kinds of phobia: *kong* and *jing*. *Kong* is a lasting, chronic reaction—for example, a phobia of cats, the dark, small spaces, etc. This type of fear creates a mood of anxiety even when the person is not directly confronted with the object of his or her fear. *Jing* is a sudden fear of something that just happened, in which case the person experiencing the fright is unsure or apprehensive about the future. (For instance, if you are walking down the street and something falls from high above almost striking you—that is a kind of sudden shock that causes unsettlement.)

TCM believes that *kong* is more disruptive to the kidney system qi while *jing* disturbs the heart system qi, including the brain. (For more about the body's systems, please see Appendix "Five Systems of the Body.") *Kong* induces a state in which qi sinks or is lowered, providing a lack of blood flow to the brain, so that it cannot perform normally. *Jing* induces a state of panic in which the person feels a loss of control. Sometimes both *jing* and *kong* happen under the same circumstance. This is a normal reaction due to the environment or situation. At that time, the body may react with raised eyebrows, eyes opened wide, looking around frantically to understand the situation. Blood rushes to big muscles and joints, away from the head to the lower half of the body, to support a possible "fight or flight" response, or the body may even become stiff as a board.

Jing usually relies on instinct and produces an immediate reaction, which, while it may be large, remains easy to get over. *Kong* can be more deep-seated and internalized. The reaction may be triggered by something that is a reminder of the fear. Although the reaction sometimes seems arbitrary or unpredictable, there is a component of the reaction of *kong* that is quite rational. An example of this type of *kong* is when a person is afraid of something that they've never personally experienced (for example, a child may develop a phobia of being bitten by a tiger after hearing a story about it). While this fear is created from fantasy, and not by experience, as is *jing*, it comes from a very real place in the mind.

Anxiety and nervousness are mild degrees of fear. For instance, before important examinations, students often get extremely anxious and nervous due to the fear of failing. A bit of stress may help performance during an examination because the heart is beating a bit faster, breathing is quicker and sometimes the arteries are full of blood, even protruding through the skin's surface. These are physical indications that the body is ready to perform, just as a hunter's pulse increases before a kill. A balance of the right kind of stress in reaction to a change is essential to the outcome of that performance or decision. Also, during a moment of loss, failure or indecision, the stress brought on by that change may allow one to move on from that situation. However, if anxiety is too deep or prolonged, it will bring negative results, especially when anxiety develops into a chronic or lasting fear.

According to Chinese medicine, *kong* will cause the kidney energy to be disharmonized, move downward, and not be held strongly by the body. The body may show signs of downward fluid movement that can manifest in reactions like easily wetting one's pants or loosing bowel moments when afraid. For some gentlemen, there may be seminal emission. Both legs become very soft and have no strength. All these symptoms can be self-diagnosed and alleviated. However, if the symptoms continue or suddenly happen uncontrollably after a week, the person should seek psychological or medical care.

Unlike *kong*, the long-lasting phobic fear that affects the kidney, *jing*, an immediate fright, usually disturbs the heart energy. The heart controls the spirit and the emotions of the person. Therefore if the heart qi is not flowing correctly, then the spirit becomes "off," flowing out of the body and causing the person to react differently or not at all. Shock may take over the body (for example, in front of a moving train or during an earthquake), paralyzing it. In many cases, these sudden experiences may be traumatic and turn into *kong*—changing from a temporary interference with the heart to a lasting phobia that affects the kidney.

My father once treated a 24-year-old woman who had experienced a very high fever that put her in a coma.

After Western medical treatment, her fever was reduced and she came out of the coma, but her sleep was never deep and sound. She developed Tourette Syndrome, constantly imagining things and repeating "someone's following me," even though she was safe at home. Every time she saw strangers, she would cry. Psychiatrists felt that she was suffering from a nervous breakdown and gave her tranquilizing medication. After treatment, she had no improvement and even developed profuse sweating as well as numbness all over the body due to the drugs, while still continuing to repeat nonsensical phrases.

When her parents brought her to my father, he indicated that she might be afraid of strangers, which usually manifests in a weak kidney, light sleep and continued repetition of nonsensical phrases, all symptoms of heart qi disorder. After regulating her kidney and heart for ten days, the woman's symptoms disappeared. Within the first five days, she started sleeping soundly, her nonsensical talking decreased, her appetite increased and bowel movements became normal. After five more days, she was talking normally, and after she had completely stopped Western medicine for two full weeks, her symptoms were cured.

Generally speaking, TCM believes people who have a temperament that is not as brave, outgoing and self-reliant are more easily frightened. A person's reaction to a situation is very much dependent on eating habits and constitution, so these indicators can make it easy for a TCM doctor to understand how to help the patient to handle emotions. For example, a lean person easily accumulates fire, loses temper and is quick to anger. More heavily-built people readily accumulate phlegm and have a temperament that is prone to fatigue and depression. There are some people who are very slim but eat a lot, as well as large people who eat very little but don't lose weight. So then, it is important to judge physical build along with eating habits, to determine temperament. Changing one's eating patterns also has the effect of changing one's temperament and reaction to different situations.

According to the *Yellow Emperor's Inner Canon*—an ancient Chinese medical text that has been the fundamental doctrinal source for TCM for more than two millennia—there are five different groups of constitution and temperament. They are based on strong or weak yin-yang energies and different movements of qi and blood. Most people have elements of more than one group but generally, if you have five or so tendencies of a group, it constitutes that you are part of that group.

Of the five groups, there is one called the *Tai Yin* Group—these people are easily frightened or chronically phobic. Their constitution is naturally more yin with very little yang. Their blood circulation is slow and sticky and their *wei qi* (or surface qi) moves slowly or is stagnant. Their yin-yang is not harmonized to have good circulation. Their skin is slightly thicker and their tendons are soft. Their temperament is usually more introverted, tending not to talk as much and preferring to be alone. They have difficulty speaking in full sentences and often hesitate. They are easily suspicious and their mental reactions are slow. They often feel victimized and apprehensive about things. Looking at their facial expressions, their mouth tends to frown and be inverted downward, and their brow is often furrowed. Their spine usually comes forward, they do not stand upright, with shoulders often hunched forward, and their action is limited. Their eyes are usually fixated on something and their minds easily wander.

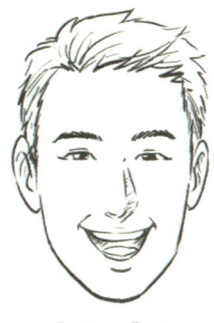
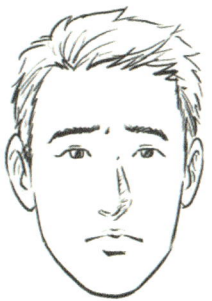

Common Face   *Tai Yin* Face

In comparative Western psychology, Kant's 1798 book *Anthropologie*, re-popularized the four different temperaments from the original text of Hippocrates, the founding father of modern medicine and precursor for Roman physician, Claudius Galen, who virtually dictated all medical theory throughout the Middle Ages. In many ways, these four also correspond to the temperaments of TCM, codified several hundred years earlier.

Humor	Physiology	Today's Dictionary Usage	MBTI™ Keirsey	Element
Sanguine	Blood	Cheerfully confident and optimistic	"sp"	Fire
Choleric	Yellow bile	Easily angered, bad tempered	"nf"	Water
Melancholic	Black bile	Depressed, melancholic, unhappy	"sj"	Earth
Phlegmatic	Phlegm	Calm, sluggish, unemotional	"nt"	Air

Kant believed the first and third were emotional temperaments, meaning their character is very much determined by how they think and approach life, while the second and fourth are actionable temperaments, meaning their emotions are very much determined by their movements and speed of action when completing a task. *Tai Yin* people may seem a bit like the melancholic temperament type. It is interesting to note that these theories, coming from different cultures and times, both use blood and phlegm as detectors of a person's constitution and temperament. According to emotional yin-yang theory, people's constitutions can be altered by working on the different organs, ultimately changing one's temperament. For *Tai Yin* types, work is done on the kidney, building essence and regulating yin and yang, and tonifying (increasing/ strengthening) the kidney yang qi. People can also incorporate lifestyle changes that will help their constitution, such as exercise outside in the sun or engaging in social activities involving sports or music. These actions may change someone who is typically *Tai Yin* to a more *Tai Yang* person. (For more information, please see Appendix "Different Constitutions and Temperaments.")

Recently, there has been a large resurgence in researching the old TCM methods of classifying different constitutions and temperaments. However, modern TCM concentrates more on classifying different constitutions according to different states of qi and blood, and deficiency of yin and yang, of which there are about six or seven depending on the school. The top institutes all agree on at least five: cold, hot, dry, damp and balanced. The constitution has two origins: congenital natural disposition and post-natal lifestyle (i.e. nature and nurture). The features of one's constitution can be detected in three areas: the physical build of the person, the functional activities of the internal body and one's psychological state. It also depends on the stage of life the person is facing, such as puberty or menopause.

Many factors influence the formation of the constitution: for instance, the parents' state of health, physically and mentally, at the time of conception, or the condition of the mother during and after the pregnancy. These two parts belong to the congenital natural disposition of one's constitution.

Most of the influence comes from our own actions and lifestyle. Of primary importance is one's diet, which we should look at on three levels. The first is basic healthy food that helps our body maintain itself on a daily basis. The second level is food for pleasure, relaxing, socializing and as a response to satisfying certain emotional moods (in moderation of course). The last is for the purpose of changing our health, reducing risks of illness, and maintaining and promoting good health. Modern nutritional sciences are now, more than ever, researching this last category as our bodies fight to stay in good health in this fast-paced and changing world. However, "functional food" or food as medicine, as we call this last category, has had 5000 years of history in Traditional Chinese Medicine.

Beyond diet, the second aspect to creating or changing a constitution is life balance—how one balances work/stress/activity with calm/quiet/reflection. Another factor is lifestyle and habits that depend on the environment (weather, pollution, seasonal changes and juxtaposition in the physical environment) and society (circle of friends, co-workers and support systems).

Marriage and conception also affect constitution. After marriage, if a couple is not initially harmonized, the partners can affect each others' constitutions. A balance of sexual activity is needed to maintain harmony in a marriage; too little or too much can affect the harmony of the body. Similarly, when women do not conceive, they may also show signs of disharmony in the body because pregnancy is a natural cycle in a woman's lifetime. A disruption in the optimal harmony in their lives, caused by not getting married, having a family situation and conceiving children, may lead to the underdevelopment of some meridian systems. Even women who decide not to breastfeed may show blockages in the liver and stomach meridians. This is due to the inability to access certain meridians connected to the action of breastfeeding and releasing milk from the body.

Illness, age and gender are also factors for one's constitution. To achieve balance and longevity, it is paramount to understand all of the many features of one's body. The core of TCM is rooted in a deep understanding of the combination of these features, in order to create a remedy or treatment plan that will bring one's health to an optimal level. These highly-individualized remedies include changing lifestyle habits and diet, and taking supplements. All food supplements and health pills come from plants, which, in turn, belong to different temperatures and flavors, and react to different meridians in the body. It is therefore vital for people to understand their constitution in order to determine which plants will work for them. (For more information on temperatures and flavors, please see Appendix "Chinese Food and Herbs.")

Remedy and Solution

Food options for treating symptoms of mild anxiety and fear

Knowing your body constitution is essential in selecting the right foods to help you manage your emotions and live a happy and high-quality life. As noted earlier, you can visit www.acherbs.com, which has a self-diagnosis banner and database summing up clinical experiences by elite TCM doctors. Through this site, you can identify your body constitution and learn about the recommended food for your individual profile.

Long-term anxiety and fear could lead to weak kidney qi, or could disturb the harmony between the kidney and heart, or the kidney and liver. Therefore functional foods are recommended that strengthen the kidney and bring harmony between kidney, heart and liver. Consequently, these foods reduce the symptoms of anxiety and stress, and help people gain more confidence.

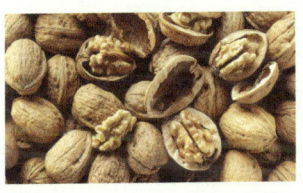

Walnut

Anxiety

Peach kernel 桃仁 10g, pistachios 15g and walnuts 15g. Eat raw or crush into a powder to take with food.
(Good for weak constitution)

Nervousness or fear, and tinnitus and hair loss

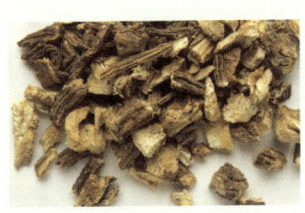

Angelica Root

Schisandra berry 五味子. Make a decoction with 5g of the berries and 10g of angelica root 当归.
(Good for cold and weak constitution)

Sesame and walnuts. Make powder of 10g of each nut, and eat on an empty stomach in the morning.

Black bean. Cook 10g with rice.

Polygonum (foti root) 首乌. Use 10g to make decoction or take 5 tablets twice a day.
(Good for hot and weak constitution)

Frequent urine and stool, seminal emission

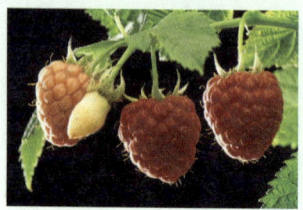
Raspberry

Semen Euryales 芡实. Cook 20g with 30g glutinous rice.
(Good for all constitutions)

Chinese raspberry 覆盆子. Eat 30g of the berries.
(Good for cold constitution)

If there is no improvement after a week, please visit a TCM doctor. For people with Lumbago, soreness around the waist and/or reproductive system, please visit a doctor immediately to find the cause.

Schisandra Berry (*wu wei zi* 五味子)

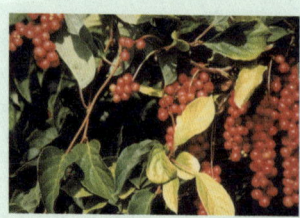
Schisandra Berry
Photograph by Dr. Alfred Kump. Courtesy of American Herbal Pharmacopoeia, Scotts Valley, CA

• **Therapeutic taste and property:** Sour, warm.
• **Function:** Astringent, calming, fortifies qi and kidney. Crude schisandra is used to stimulate the production of fluids, clear deficiency of fire, and relieve cough.
• **Application:** Calms the spirit, used for insomnia, palpitations and poor memory.
• **Usage and Dosage:** 2-6g is used in decoction for eating. 1-3g of the powder is swallowed after meal.
• **Contraindication:** Schisandra is contraindicated if there is an excess of exterior and interior heat and in the early stages of cough and rashes.

Recipe:

Chicken Soup

- **Ingredients:** One whole free-range chicken, three pieces of ginger, three spring onions, two teaspoons of rice wine or white wine, 3-5g salt.
- **Preparation:** Wash chicken and chop into 2cm×6cm pieces. Put chicken into earthenware pot (or Chinese clay pot), and add water to a level of 3-5cm over chicken. Cook with high heat until boiling, then add ginger and wine, and boil for 2 minutes. Reduce heat and stew for 1 hour, adding the onion and salt near the end.
- **Function:** Chicken is sweet and warm in flavor and temperature. Adding wine, ginger and spring onion can increase body energy, balance the internal organs' yin and yang, increase vitality, and control and reduce anxiety and fear.

Self-Acupressure Point

Hundred Convergences (Baihui 百会)

Location: At the top of skull, on the middle line of the head, at the crossing of the line that runs vertically intersecting the nose with the line that runs from ear to ear.

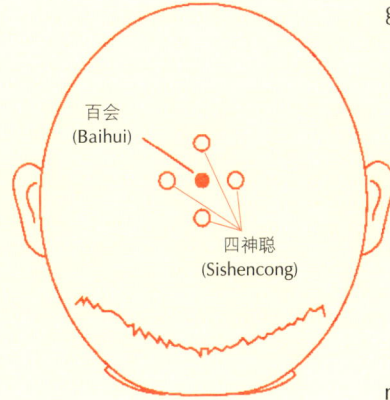

Function: Subdues liver yang and extinguishes liver wind, strengthens the ascending function of the spleen and wakes senses.

Indication: Headache at top of head, mental disorder of sinking yang, vertigo, and aphasia.

Method: Press in clockwise and counterclockwise circles for five minutes. Using the palm to massage the Baihui area helps stabilize the spirit. It prevents insomnia, poor memory and mental disorders.

Chapter 2
Managing Emotions through the Five Elements: the Heart System

心者，君主之官，神明出焉。
　　　　　　　　——《黄帝内经》
Xin zhe, jun zhu zhi guan, shen ming chu yan.

The heart is the "emperor" organ and dominates mental activities.

—*Yellow Emperor's Inner Canon*

The *jun zhu* or emperor, the heart, is in control of the entire body's physical and psychological functions. It is the storehouse of the spirit. The broader meaning of the spirit refers to one's activities throughout a lifetime, all of which are part of a connected framework. People can only comprehend the complexities of inner vitality and health through outer representations, all of which TCM calls the "spirit": complexion, expression of the eyes, movements and speech. The more narrow meaning of spirit relates to a person's consciousness and mental activity: How one contemplates life, the individual's emotional state and also the quality of sleep. These are the major functions of the heart according to TCM.

亢则害，承乃制。
——《黄帝内经》

Kang ze hai, cheng nai zhi.

Extreme conditions are very harmful, but the effects can be remedied if we find the right ways to restrain them.

—*Yellow Emperor's Inner Canon*

In the Five Elements theory, there are two relationships between one element and another: How one element can generate or produce another (water generates wood, for instance) and how one extinguishes or controls the other (water controls fire). On a large scale, this relates to the natural balance in the universe, and on a smaller scale, to functions of the human body, which is a microcosm of the universe. Damage is caused if one of the Five Elements is in excess, just as if you over-water plants, they soon wilt. This is called *kang ze hai*.

The second half of the proverb describes what happens when an excess of some elements arises: A counter force will start to rise and restore balance between the two forces. Eventually, the body system achieves overall harmony. The five major *zang* organs (heart, lung, kidney, liver, spleen) are associated with the Five Elements. Their balance is important to a person's metabolic function and psychological state. Disruption of that balance brings about disruption of good health.

In TCM, there are seven emotions to be considered: joy, anger, worry, longing, sadness, fear and fright (shock). These emotions, which are reactions to our environment, affect us psychologically and physiology. Our body and soul are closely linked and influenced by one another. Every emotion has beneficial and harmful effects on the human body, so we need to be familiar with the harmful effects and how to control them. Knowledge and awareness is the first step towards understanding, from which we can embark on effective change.

Now let us begin with "joy."

Case Story

The Ming dynasty Classic *The Unofficial History of the Scholars (Rulin waishi* 儒林外史) tells of a person named Fan Jin who was busy preparing for high-level candidacy for the Mandarin examinations. Though his family was very poor and he was without a stable job, Fan Jin received permission from a well-to-do local pig butcher to marry his daughter, as Fan Jin was a reliable, honest and faithful person who was always trying to better his lot. His mother and wife were constantly depending on his father-in-law for support, making Fan Jin more determined to take the examinations to increase his economic and social standing.

For many years he took the test, always only testing to the lowest level, and still having difficulty finding a good job. Then, one year, his tutor told him that he believed Fan Jin could test to the high-level of *ju ren*, a revered title that would ensure employment and a better future for his family. Although he lacked confidence after many failures, the tutor's encouragement won him over. He ended up taking the exam, and afterward, even going about daily chores he felt more accomplished.

One day at the market, Fan Jin was suddenly accosted by a neighbor: "Go home! There is a group of people from the exam committee carrying a banner

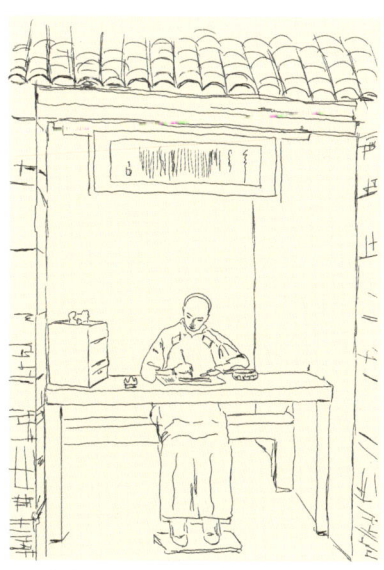

Mandarin Examination

down the street to your house. It says you've received the highest honor of *ju ren*! Quickly go home to receive it!" Fan Jin initially took this as a jest, but after much persuasion, he finally went home to see what the ruckus was all about.

Upon returning home and seeing the banner congratulating him on passing the highest level of examinations, his demeanor switched to an almost unrecognizable state. He clapped his hands uncontrollably and guffawed like a madman, repeating many times, "Ha ha! Fantastic! I made it!" Suddenly he fell backwards and clenched his teeth, losing consciousness. After coming to again, he stood up, began to clap his hands and laughed loudly, repeating, "I made it! I made it!" As he ran out the door, everyone was frightened and unable to stop him.

He continued in this ridiculous state to everyone's dismay until finally, a person with traditional medical knowledge had an idea, "Quick! Who is Fan Jin afraid of?" The townspeople mentioned his father-in-law, and then the person proceeded to reverse the effects. He told the father-in-law to yell at Fan Jin and slap him hard across the face, telling him that he had actually NOT passed the examinations, that it was all a hoax. While this method was relatively severe, it served to snap Fan Jin back into reality, so much so that once he recovered his breath, he vomited phlegm and after a few moments became very calm and returned to normal.

Analysis

In TCM, happiness is considered a positive yang emotion that tends to flow upward and outward, internally relaxing qi and blood. It can help balance emotions, open the mind and heart, and regulate the body's energy and blood circulation. It helps in balancing physiological and mental states. As an emotion, it relates to the heart organ system and the fire element. (See Appendix for an explanation of the Five Systems.)

According to TCM, the heart governs the spirit-mind, which refers to the clarity of the consciousness and the strength of mental and emotional faculties. In Western physiology, these are considered functions of the brain, but in TCM they are variously attributed to the organs. The heart system is considered particularly important in this context.

In dealing with an excess of any emotion in TCM, it is important to consider the situation, environment, symptoms and constitution of the person before remedying, as they all play an important factor in balancing the right elements.

In Western medicine, when we are "happy" emotionally, physiologically the central nervous system decreases the production of chemicals that cause negative emotions in the brain. When happy, the drive for action and productivity is increased, and the brain is stimulated. Even through difficulty, your coping abilities are heightened. This is why remedies that focus on increasing levels of happiness are often used to alleviate diseases such as depression and anxiety. Comedy is a universal medicine, and while most of us would like to increase our happiness in daily life, excessive happiness can actually make one act abnormally or feel unbalanced, as seen in our story above.

TCM theory states that there is a balanced line between all emotions, positive or negative. Everything is

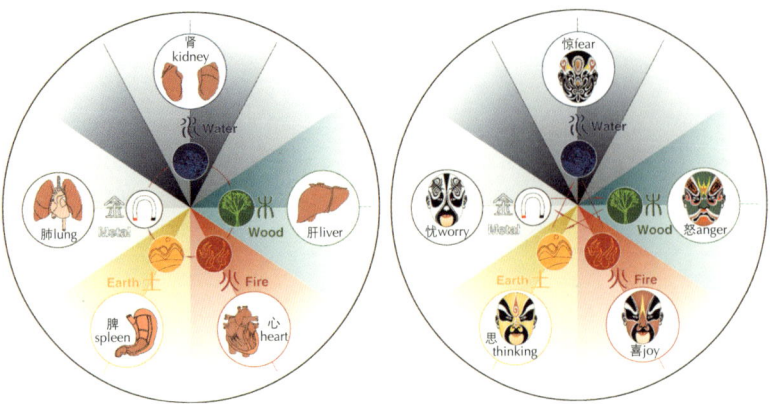

Diagram of the Five Elements

better in harmony and anything excessive can lead to an imbalance. Sudden happiness or excessive happiness for long periods of time can strain our individual coping abilities and can produce a negative effect. This was the case with Fan Jin.

Another example can be seen through Olympic ice-skater Dan Jansen in the 1994 Olympics. Previously, he always won silver or bronze medals, never winning the gold. During the Winter Olympic 1000m speed skating event, he promised his sister the gold, knowing she was terminally ill. This drive brought him the gold that year. His wife became overly ecstatic, fainted and was carried out of the stadium by ambulance.

There are records of similar cases where excessive happiness even leads to death. For example, every year, there are a few deaths during the World Cup, which in

TCM would be related to heart failure, stroke or sudden attacks brought on by an over-elated feeling.

Under the Five Elements theory, excessive happiness (sudden or long-term) can cause the heart system to be out of balance. In mild cases, people have a lack of concentration, insomnia, palpitations, and sometimes cannot control their mental state. In severe cases, it can cause the energy of the heart to spread out, dispersing energy control, and causing a dangerous separation of yin and yang energy. This can lead to fainting, nervous breakdown, and even heart failure and death. In Chinese medicine this is called, *guo xi shang xin* 过喜伤心, or "Over Happiness Affecting the Heart." (For an explanation of the Five Elements theory and its effect on the organs, please see Appendix.)

There is a belief in TCM that a disharmony in the organs can also result in unusual emotional behavior. Normally, deficient heart qi causes sadness, while excessive heart qi can cause madness and over-stimulation from happiness. By regulating and strengthening the qi in the organs, you can bring emotions back to a balanced state.

In Western psychology, there are two minds: the rational and the irrational. These also need a certain harmony. The rational mind has often been equated with the brain, and the irrational mind, the soul. Sudden excessive emotion can cause the central nervous system to short-circuit, causing a jolt of fear, sudden shouting or release of tension, fainting or some other kind of physiological reaction. During that reaction time, the irrational mind—in particular, the limbic-amyglada (*bian yuan xi tong–xing ren he* 边缘系统–杏仁核) or triune brain, sometimes known as the reptilian brain—sends stimulated signals, preparing the whole body for action. During the momentary lapse during the short-circuiting, the rational mind—and in particular, the New cortex (xin pi zhi 新皮质)—doesn't get a chance to process the overall response as a beneficial or harmful one. Instead, the irrational mind responds quickly, without proper judgment, creating a primal "fight or flight" reaction to the situation. This was the case with Fan Jin.

In our story, it was Fan Jin's father-in-law who remedied his case. He did this by slapping him, shouting and making him frightened. Why is it that fear can harmonize excessive happiness? According to the Five Elements theory, over-happiness belongs to the fire element and fear belongs to water. In the natural universe, water controls fire, and therefore a simple switch in Fan Jin's emotional state by inducing fear (water) controlled his over-happiness (fire). This is called TCM Psychological Therapy. (See Appendix for more on how the Five Elements theory is used to manage emotions.)

The factors that induce emotional fluctuations are various. Apart from an important examination, as in the case of Fan Jin, any unexpected life event can potentially cause a long-term imbalance. As I write this, there were over 4000 children orphaned in one day when China's Sichuan Province was hit by a massive earthquake, television broadcasts showing their frightened faces, crying and state of shock from the situation that changed their fate within minutes. If people cannot efficaciously adjust and adapt, they can suffer long-term emotional damage.

Apart from natural disasters or traumatic events, sociological factors can also affect one's emotions. In the case of Fan Jin, his excessive happiness was not caused just by achieving success but also from the imbalance brought about by his sudden new fame and fortune.

Depression is a common emotion when people retire or fall from high positions of wealth and status, losing their titles and previous positions in society and therefore affecting their belief of self-worth. (Cases of depression from physiological reasons can be found in Chapter 6.)

On the flip side, excessive happiness is possible when jumping into new fortune. How many times do we hear of people fainting when winning the lottery or scoring the jackpot? For those with a strong constitution, handling these emotions can be done with grace. Those with a fickle constitution are usually affected more easily.

Happiness is an emotion that can certainly bring many positive effects. Therefore, it is important to judge if one is experiencing regular or excessive happiness. If happiness brings a high but overall stable mood in daily life—marked by good sleep and emotions—then this is considered positive, encouraging happiness. If there is a sudden onset of nervousness, palpitations, difficulty concentrating, excessive smiling or disturbed sleep, then this is a case of over-happiness.

It is easy to change these levels back to normal by oneself, with attention to sleep and self-awareness. Taking actions to help others and concentrating on matters that don't bring on that level of elation are all ways to alleviate mild over-happiness. If happiness becomes uncontrollable, marked by smiling at awkward times, suddenly fainting or becoming mentally or physically separate (for instance, regressing to childhood or acting strangely), then medical consultation is necessary to manage recovery.

Remedy and Solution

Food options for treating symptoms of mild over-happiness

Disturbances of heart qi and blood, and imbalance of heart yin and yang, will lead to emotional imbalance. Since the heart is the organ system that controls spirit and emotion, to treat this emotional imbalance, we need to first regulate the heart.

Difficulty sleeping, insomnia, dream-disturbed sleep

Chrysanthemum. Mix 2 flowers with 150ml boiling water for tea.

Chamomile leaf. Use 2g to make tea. Drink 30 minutes before sleep.
(Good for hot constitution or in summer)

Honey. Take 1 teaspoon to mix with 80ml warm milk.

Lingzhi mushroom 灵芝. Use 6-9g to make decoction, take twice a day after meal. Drink 30 minutes before sleep.
(Good for cold constitution or in winter)

Tiger lily buds 黄花菜. Take 20g dried and soak in water for 10 minutes, then cut in half, make soup and add honey (optional). Drink 150ml 1 hour before sleep.

Boiled fresh peanuts. Make decoction with leaf (50g). Drink the liquid (75ml) and eat nuts (5-10g) in afternoon or evening time.
(Good for people with blood deficiencies or those recovering from illness or a recent operation)

Managing Emotions through the Five Elements: the Heart System

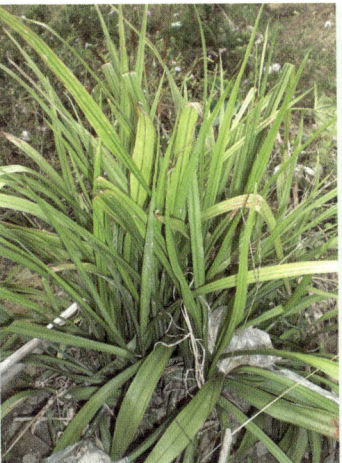

Tiger Lily Buds (Huang Hua Cai),
Photograph by Yao Yingzhi

Heart palpitations from being alarmed and vexed

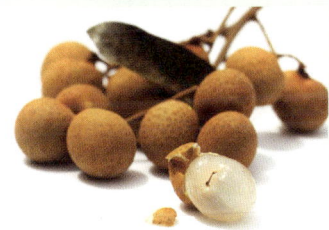

Longan Fruit

Longan (dragon eyes) fruit 龙眼 and jujube (Chinese red date) 红枣. Eat 30g of fresh longan fruit or 15g of dry, and 6 dry jujube pieces a day. Eat fruits or make soup.
(Good for people with qi and blood deficiencies and cold constitution or during the winter)

Aloe vera 芦荟 juice or yogurt. Eat 200ml once a day before meal.

Oyster meat 牡蛎. Eat 120g of fresh oysters or drink 50ml of decoction made from 30g cooked dry oyster shell.
(Good for people with hot constitution or in summer)

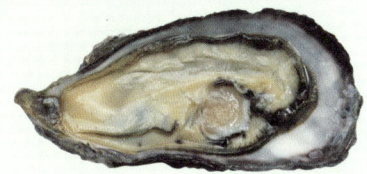

Oyster

43

Semen Ziziphus Spinosa (*suan zao ren* 酸枣仁)

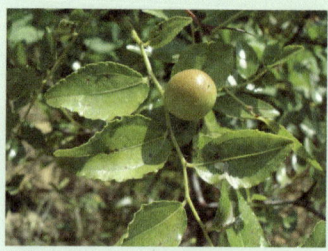

Semen Ziziphus Sopinosa
Photograph Courtesy of
Herbasinica, Shenyang, China

• **Therapeutic taste and property:** Sweet and sour, neutral.
• **Function:** Nourish the heart, benefit the liver, tranquilize the mind and stop excessive perspiration.
• **Application:** Indicated for insomnia and vexation. It is commonly used as a medicine to treat restlessness from various causes, particularly nutrition-deficient syndrome. These symptoms are caused by deficiency of heart-blood and liver-blood. It can also be used to treat spontaneous perspiration and night sweating.
• **Usage and Dosage:** 9-15g is used in decoction for drinking. 1.5-3g of the powder is swallowed before bed.

Recipe:

Chrysanthemum Tea

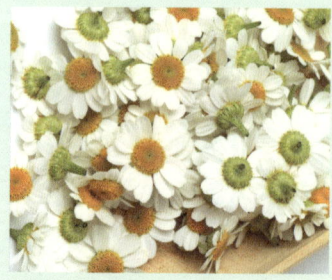

Chrysanthemum Flower

• **Ingredients:** 2 chrysanthemum flowers, 150ml boiling water, honey.
• **Preparation:** Put chrysanthemum flowers into cup then add 150ml boiling water. Keep lid on for 5 minutes then add honey (optional).
• **Function:** Dispels excessive heat, relaxes mind and encourages good sleep, especially making falling sleep easier.

Self-Acupressure Point

Water Trough (Shuigou 水沟)

Location: Above the upper lip, in the crease, one third of the distance from the base of the nasal septum to the red skin of the upper lip on the midline.

Function: Promotes resuscitation and opens the orifices. Clears Heat.

Indication: Treat mental disordens hysteria, coma and faint.

Method: For suddenly fainting, it is best not to change the position of the person but you can try pressing on the spot. Press in counterclockwise circles for 1 minute.

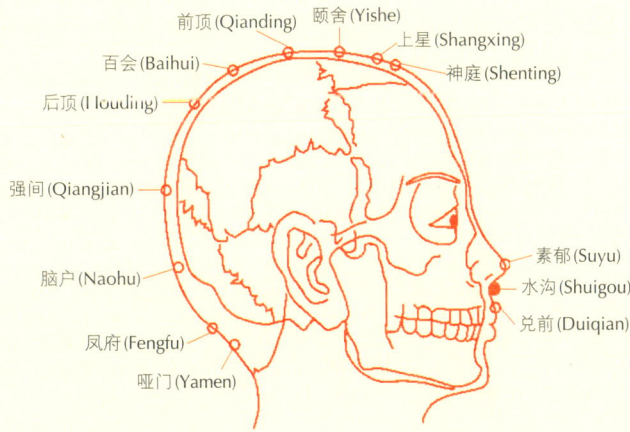

Chapter 3
Managing Emotions through Yin-Yang Theory: the Lung System

肺者，相傅之官，治节出焉。
——《黄帝内经》

Fei zhe, xiang fu zhi guan, zhi jie chu yan.

The lung is the management organ and is responsible for governing and regulating [energy, blood and body fluid circulation].

—*Yellow Emperor's Inner Canon*

The lung is considered the "Prime Minister" of the body, receiving all messages from the heart and administering these signals throughout the whole body, especially producing, controlling and regulating the body's qi through breath. It controls the circulation of blood and regulates the body's metabolism of fluid, establishing the balance needed for good health.

万物负阴而抱阳,冲气以为和。

——老子

Wan wu fu yin er bao yang, chong qi yi wei he.

The characteristics of all things in the universe have yin and yang. Yin and yang reach dynamic balance through movement.

—**Laozi**

All things and phenomena in the universe contain a part of yin and a part of yang. The direct meaning of this quote from Laozi, the famous Chinese philosopher, is for one to carry the yin on one's back, holding the yang on one's front. Through movement and changes, these two essences achieve a dynamic and relative equilibrium. A balanced attitude and mood as well as positive-minded and open-hearted disposition are based on the movements of energy and blood caused by the dynamics of yin and yang.

Case Story 1

Mr. Shen, the CEO of an architecture and design company, lost his wife recently. They were very close, and since her death, he has not been the same, suffering from extreme sadness ever since. He keeps his wife's room as if she was still alive and locks himself in the house after work. Coming back home, he yearns to talk to her, losing interest in activities, learning new things, meeting new people or exercising. His sleep is never deep, and every day, he loses more and more energy.

Case Story 2

Helen, a company secretary, lost all of her financial savings due to the bankruptcy of a regional bank. She had put all of her money into one bank account, including her personal pension and healthcare savings for many years. The bank was only able to return ten percent of her losses and since then, she has not been the same, finding it difficult to breathe, feeling pressure on her chest and experiencing shallow breathing, as well as suffering from a constant worry about her health and future. She no longer likes to go out and says, "This is not the life I want; I don't feel like myself any more."

Analysis

The first case reflects the loss of a loved one in the family. Based on TCM yin and yang theory, sadness is

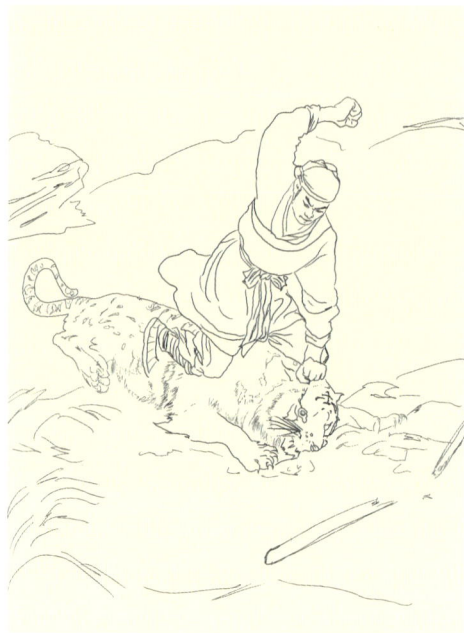

An Ancient Chinese
Fighting a Tiger

known as the yin of emotions, while happiness is the yang of emotions. Excess yin energy holds and stores emotions internally and is often associated with introverted thought that spirals inwards. Most of our body's functions slow down and our mental capacity, along with our ability to be affectionate and outwardly warm, diminish. The emotion of happiness has the opposite effect, causing us to be open and able to look at things from a different viewpoint.

No matter whether the emotion is yin or yang, there should be a balance of both. Even though yin emotion seems to have draining effects, it is only detrimental when yin qi is in excess. In early stages of human development, excessive yin energy was necessary for the development of what is sometimes called the R-complex or Reptilian brain, the part responsible for basic survival responses.

Sadness is a natural human emotion that needs to

be felt, and withstanding loss and internalizing emotions can bring their own benefits. Sad people usually decline invitations to go out or to partake in social occasions, allowing the body to be more "at rest" and slowing down its metabolism. It is a time of reflection and assimilating thoughts to begin anew. It is also a time for spiritual grounding, a time for dealing with emotions, a time to heal and accumulate strength to move on. In prehistoric times, humans needed times of sadness as a security system to prevent further loss and damage in their lives. People would use these times of reflection to determine how to better secure their livelihoods and develop more advanced defensive techniques.

However, being stuck in a state of sadness can induce depression and even make people lose the will to live. In TCM, this prolonged sadness can damage the lung, the organ system that handles sad emotions. An existing weakened lung state can produce an exacerbated effect. Deeper and longer sadness can consume lung qi, and people with pre-existing lung qi deficiency cannot handle even mild sadness.

Your basic constitution affects how you deal with a situation of loss—either as a victim or with a positive outlook. Those with stronger constitutions (positive outlook) can withstand certain levels of loss by learning and gaining experience from it, whereas those with weaker constitutions (negative outlooks/victims) tend to give in to their physical state and more easily become ill or unbalanced, feeling consumed by the situation. (For related symptoms, see Chapter 1.)

As sadness causes lung energy consumption, it easily leads to symptoms such as crying, fatigue, shortness of breath, loss of appetite, middle-qi (spleen-stomach qi) deficiency, a loss of energy in the voice, a diminished spirit, and may even induce mechanical deficiencies in the lung, such as tuberculosis and bronchitis. In severe cases, it leads to depression.

As sadness is a yin emotion, TCM doctors use yang methods to harmonize and balance it. Specifically, TCM psychologists use happiness to control sadness. Even if the happiness is not real, they will select something relevant to the patient, and create unsuspected moments of happiness to resolve the illness brought on by sadness.

One example can be taken from a Ming dynasty story. A woman's husband left for business and disappeared for two years with no word. She suspected something terrible had happened to him or that he met another woman. From longing and worrying about him, she became severely depressed. Doctors knew they couldn't cure her only with herbs and eventually said, "Your husband has been found and is coming back in a few days. He's healthy and very successful after two years of hard work. You will be reunited and he will bring lots of fortune home." Even though the doctor was lying, he wanted to make her suddenly happy.

The doctor also asked the servants to mess up the house, break household goods and ruin the bed sheets. As the woman was a tidy person, this made her angry, bringing out all the stuck energy in her body. This surge of energy caused her to cough up large amounts of phlegm and she became very tired. The next day, she was back to normal.

Two of the Five Elements were used in handling this case: Happiness (Fire) controlled Sadness/Worry (Metal) in the short term, and Anger (Wood) controlling Missing/Longing (Earth) changed her qi balance for the long term. These two methods of inducing opposite emotions through Five Element theory can harmonize stagnant qi in the body and make it relatively balanced again.

TCM uses yin-yang theory to analyze and group different patterns of conditions caused by emotions. Rooted in Chinese philosophy, over-happiness is believed to disturb yang qi in the body. Excessive sadness is believed to disturb yin qi in the body. Anger, worry, depression, longing, failure and fear all influence our body qi, blood and overall yin and yang in different ways.

TCM identified yin and yang patterns of schizophrenia long before Western medicine. TCM theory also observes that excess yang can bring about pathological change and may lead towards the following symptoms: loud and disruptive noise making, propensity to want to hurt other people or animals, anger-induced actions and movements, a tendency to over-reaction or loss of patience, hyperactivity, and selfish and narcissistic action. Excess yin may lead to manic-depression, with these observed symptoms: disinterest in conversation, illogical speech or thought, lethargy and inappropriate smiling.

Yang qi is a kind of positive, affirmative energy that goes "up and out" to make our energy strong, proactive and harmonious. Negative emotions are more complicated; some make yang energy stagnant, or cause it to move upward (in the direction of anger), face inward (diminished energy, sadness, depression), downward (uncontrollable fear) or down and outward (shock).

To fully understand the symptoms, it is important to identify not only the excess amount of yin or yang that affects a person but also to first recognize the person's constitution and patterns of behavior. So, in TCM we use opposing methods to balance the movement of qi, depending on their origin and related patterns. (For more information, please see Appendix "Yin-Yang Theory.")

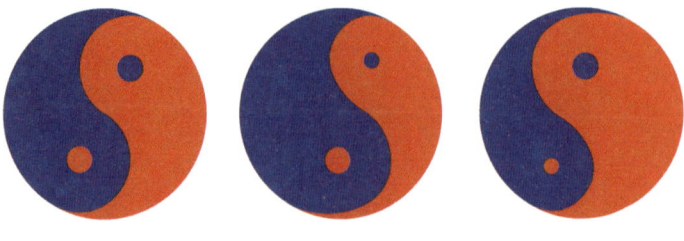

Yin-Yang Diagram

Generally speaking, when people have been diagnosed with a yang pattern emotional disorder, having a bit of yin food can control an excess of yang energy. If they have been diagnosed with a yin pattern of emotional disorder, having yang foods (particularly spices) usually helps. The section that follows contains some recipes and acupressure points to deal with sadness and worry.

It is important to note that certain constitutions and temperaments can make emotions very delicate to handle. One example in Chinese history is Lin Daiyu from the classic *A Dream of Red Mansions*, a tale of love, infidelity, familial responsibilities, succession of power and ultimately, jealousy. The female protagonist, Lin, has a weak constitution and temperament: feeling fatigue and low endurance, lacking strength in muscles and joints, and easily catching a cold or reacting to a change in weather. Her facial color is paler, with no brightness in her skin or eyes. There is great depth that goes into the description of her weak constitution and physical state, which ultimately gives the reader an idea of her character and ability to handle emotional situations. Emotionally, weak constitutions tend to worry more, are easily tearful and get hurt emotionally by others' comments. They rarely smile brightly and tend to be more quiet and shy. In *A Dream of*

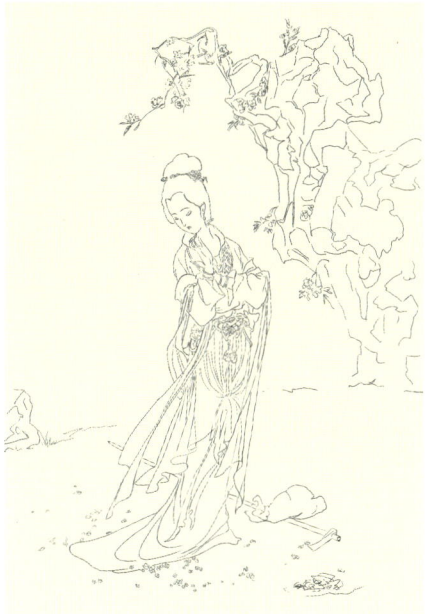

Lin Daiyu

Red Mansions, Lin was easily hurt for a few days by simple jokes or jesting criticisms from her love. One chapter is even dedicated to her crying over flowers falling from trees, which she buried in the ground.

One's constitution, influenced through congenital and environmental factors, determines physical or emotional reactions and how they should be treated. It is also interesting to note three distinct levels of emotional state in TCM: the basic reaction on the immediate level (situational), the seven emotions mentioned in this book, and one's overall spiritual state or personality, or the attitude resulting from all the things accumulated in a lifetime. It is via these three levels of awareness, along with a basic understanding of the person's constitution, by which the best method to balance the individual is determined by Chinese Medicine Theory.

Remedy and Solution

Food options for treating symptoms of mild over-worry, sadness and grief

Long-term sadness or worry will lead to deficiencies of both lung energy and yin. Sometimes weakness of heart qi, or phlegm blockage in the chest or facial sinus, makes people worry easily. Therefore, strengthening chest energy and removing phlegm blockages will help people become more optimistic.

Some general advice for people who worry easily is that eating more beans, nuts and fish to tonify lung and heart energy. Recommended foods include black beans, soy beans, pumpkin seeds and salmon. For people with lung yin weakness (thirst and dry throat), add lily bulb and tiger lily buds.

These remedies are advisable for people who often feel shortness of breath, are easily cold or spontaneously sweat. They need to take a broad range of foods, absorb all the nutrition from vegetables, neutral and warm fruits (for example, grapes, oranges and apples), grains, beans and meat (to get proteins and good fat), and a broad, balanced range of vitamins and minerals.

Sorrow, forgetfulness

Fresh Chinese yam 山药. Once a day, stir-fry 50g along with 10g of black fungus 黑木耳 or Chinese lettuce root 莴苣, or make soup with any vegetables. Or boil for 5 minutes then eat as salad with

Lettuce

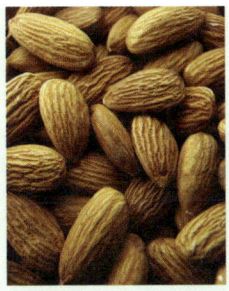
Almond

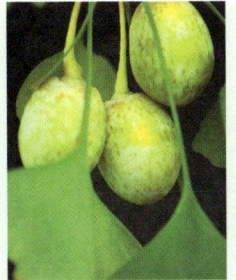
Gingko Nut

lettuce. You can also add 30g of dried yam powder to yogurt.
(Good for all constitutions)

Shortness of breath or cough, asthma, accumulation of phlegm

Gingko nut 白果. Boil 8 nuts for 2 minutes, take shell off and eat the nuts.

Polygala root (Radix Polygalae) 远志 or almond 杏仁. Take 6g daily.
(Good for weak and cold constitutions)

Ophiopogon tuber 麦冬 (亦称麦门冬) or lily bulb 百合. Cook 10g daily as dessert.

Momordica fruit 罗汉果. Slice 5g and make as a tea. Also prevents dry mouth and hoarseness and treats sore throat.
(Good for hot constitution)

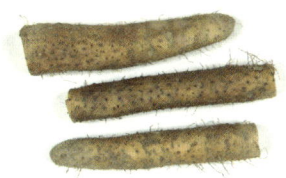
Chinese Yam

Spontaneous sweat

White fungus 银耳 (edible fungus) 100g, 15 pieces jujubes (Chinese red date) 红枣, Chinese yam 山药 30g. Soak fungus and dates in water for 1 hour, then bring to a boil and stew for 1 hour. Peel the skin off the yams and cut into small cubes. Add to fungus/date soup and boil for 15 minutes. Add honey (optional).
(Good for weak or normal constitutions)

Radix Polygalae (*yuan zhi* 远志)

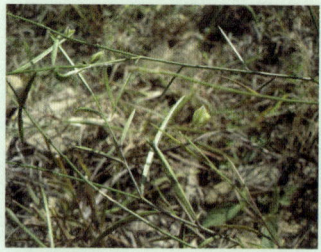

Radix polygalae
Photograph Courtesy of Herbasinica, Shenyang, China

- **Therapeutic Taste and Property:** Pungent and bitter, slightly warm.
- **Function:** Calm the mind, eliminate phlegm and dissipate carbuncles.
- **Application:**
  1. Treat irritability, palpitation due to fright, insomnia and amnesia.
  2. Treat mental confusion, absent-mindedness and epilepsy due to fright.
  3. For cough with excessive phlegm that is difficult to expectorate.
  4. For large carbuncles and pain of the breast, it can be used no matter whether the syndrome is due to cold or heat, asthenia or sthenia. It can be ground into powder that is taken alone with millet wine, or that is mixed for external application.
- **Usage and Dosage:** 3-10g is used in decoction for drinking.
- **Contraindication:** It is used with caution in patients who suffer from ulcer and gastritis.

Recipe:

Licorice, Jujube and Wheat Decoction

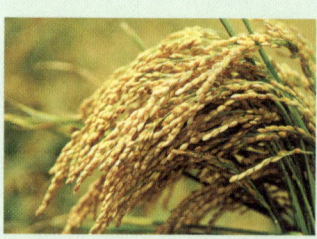

Wheat

- **Ingredients:** Licorice 甘草10g, common wheat小麦30g, 10 jujubes 红枣 (Chinese red date).
- **Preparation:** Add water to a level of 5cm over dry ingredients and soak in earthenware pot for 1 hour. Bring to boil then simmer for 30 minutes. Pour off liquid (reserve for later use), then add 500 ml water and cook for second time. Mix 2nd batch of liquid with reserved liquid, and drink half in the morning and half in the evening.
- **Function:** For hysteria, depression, insomnia, nervous breakdown or menopause symptoms caused by heart and lung yin deficiency.

Self-Acupressure Point

Hall of Impression (Yintang 印堂)

Location: Between the eyebrows, on the anterior midline at the center of the glabella.
Function: Quiets the spirit and calms the mind.
Indication: Treats childhood fears, high blood pressure, frontal headaches, heavy-headedness, trigeminal neuralgia, insomnia.
Method: Press clockwise for 25 circles, counterclockwise for 25 circles, ending with wiping 5 times to relax.

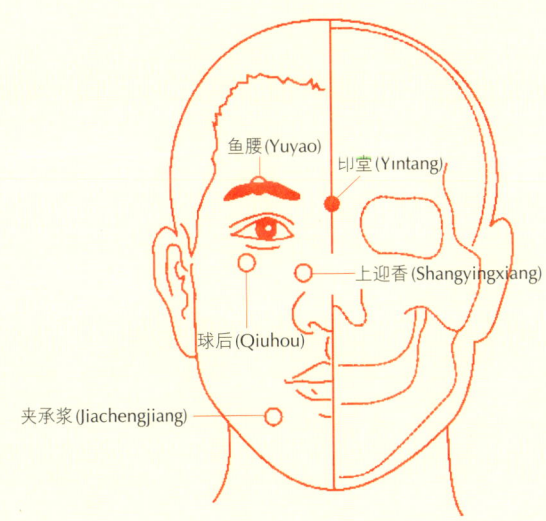

Chapter 4
Managing the Complex Emotional Cycle: the Liver System

肝者，将军之官，罢极之本，主疏泄。
——《黄帝内经》

Gan zhe, jiang jun zhi guan, pi ji zhi ben, zhu shu xie.

The liver is the planning organ in charge of mood, causing ups and downs. The liver governs dispersing and regulating qi.

—*Yellow Emperor's Inner Canon*

The liver is the "General" of the whole body. It regulates a person's mood, including feelings of depression or excitement. The liver controls the inherent facilities of the body such as eating or reproductive urges.

月始生，则血气始精，卫气始行；
月郭满，则血气实，肌肉坚；
月郭空，则肌肉减，经络虚，卫气去，形独居。是以因天时而调血气也。
——《黄帝内经》

Yue shi sheng, ze xue qi shi jing, wei qi shi xing; yue kuo man, ze xue qi shi; ji rou jian; yue kuo kong, ze ji rou jian, jing luo xu, wei qi qu, xing du ju. Shi yi yin tian shi er tiao xue qi ye.

When the moon begins to show a crescent, blood and qi circulate smoothly and defensive qi strengthens. When the moon is full, blood and qi are superabundant and the muscles are strongest. When the moon wanes, the muscles become weak, the channels and collaterals [qi and blood] are at their weakest; the defensive qi is deficient although the physical body shows no change. That is why blood and qi should be regulated with cyclical variation.

—*Yellow Emperor's Inner Canon*

Traditionally, the Chinese have believed that a waxing moon correlates with changes in the environment and the human body. The development of energy and blood also mimic the moon, growing more and more full and active. Defensive energy also increases and flows more smoothly. Then once the moon is completely full, energy and blood nourishment reach levels that are optimal for each individual. Outwardly, this manifests in the physicality of the body with visible signs of strength. When the moon begins to wane, physical strength diminishes. The meridian energy and blood get weaker (again, relative to the person), and there is a diminished spirit, even though the physical structure of the body looks the same.

According to TCM, all emotions, whether active or calm, are contingent on the quality and quantity of energy and blood as well as their relative harmony in the body. This provides a mechanism for people to understand the inevitable changes of the body on a monthly basis. That is why our emotional cycles are 28 to 30 days long. Change happens every day. Noticing this change and understanding it will prevent irregular or excessive emotional changes.

Case Story

A patient had a health problem for years, which neither Western allopathic nor homeopathic medicine alleviated. A hormonal imbalance had very bad repercussions on her mood, body and concentration, and provoked extreme tiredness. She reached a point where she felt she could not take it anymore, so she turned to Traditional Chinese Medicine for answers.

When the patient was young, she was prescribed Progesterone but stopped due to the heavy retention of water that caused a weight gain of about six kilograms. Also, the medication did not resolve the most important issue: feeling comfortable with herself, with a sense of peace and calm. Three years ago, she consulted a gynecologist who prescribed Primrose Evening Oil (1000g, three times daily). It worked a little but not significantly.

The most frustrating issues were the mood swings, fatigue, pent-up aggression and inability to concentrate, which really affected her daily life and ability to work. The changes happened suddenly and always around two weeks before her period. The patient felt as if she never got a break, continuously retaining water and gaining weight. As she grew older, she also noticed a propensity to be more sensitive to things, crying easily—a trait she never had in the past.

The patient did not wish to take a birth control pill, which had consistently been recommended by many doctors, as she believed these are artificial hormones that would not allow her body to manage its own state naturally, and therefore would not provide a long-term solution.

Analysis

In TCM, there is a phenomenon called "The Complex Emotional Cycle," and it is made up of two parts: the natural cycle of emotions and the hormonal menstrual cycle. These two cycles both influence mood, and, obviously, affect men and women differently, as men only have one of the cycles. It is the interaction of both that causes a tendency for women to have more noticeable mood swings during different times in the cycle. (See chapter 6 for more examples.)

In TCM, there are three varying degrees of one's emotional state during the menstrual cycle: mild, medium and extreme. Generally speaking, most women will have one to three days of emotional changes, or noted imbalance, pre-menstruation. These symptoms are considered mild if they don't include depression, anxiety or feeling tired with headaches. It's easy to feel slightly down and tense, lack concentration and have tenderness of the breasts, slight fullness in the abdomen, and weakness in the lower back. This is a common condition for women pre-menstruation and the way to alleviate the symptoms is to take it easy, handling stress and fatigue to return to a balanced state.

The normal menstrual cycle is 28 to 30 days long or can vary between 25 to 35 days. The period is usually three to seven days long. The quantity of blood should be 70 to 120 milliliters, with an average of 100 milliliters lost. The color should be fresh, bright red or dark-red with a half day of small clots over the first and second days. TCM emphasizes that special care should take place during this time; it is important to keep warm, include warming foods in one's diet, get enough rest and work less to decrease one's stress.

In the second, or medium degree, these symptoms accumulate for a longer period of time (four to seven days, before or during menstruation), and are more pronounced, possibly including abdominal pain, water retention, cravings for sweets, being easily moved to tears or depression, or even general aggressiveness or loss of temper. Physical symptoms may include headaches; breasts that are tender or become full or painful, or even have lumps; painful cramps; heaviness of the limbs; lower backaches; and a type of muscle-aching fatigue. If symptoms are no longer helped by the daily care of a good diet and relaxation, then an imbalance has occurred.

In order to assess the condition, women should note what is happening to them for the first month, not immediately consulting a doctor. The reasons for the symptoms could be over-work, outside stress or a lack of attention to diet; many cases have been due to excessive dieting or eating overly cold foods. There could be a possible change in birth control methods. The blood may be slightly scanty and take longer to show fresh blood, or menstruation may either be delayed or arrive early. With adjustments in life, these symptoms are all easily prone to change—it is important for each individual to understand her own situation.

The patient is in the third (extreme) degree if more than three of the above symptoms feel uncontrollable over seven days. Irritable and violent feelings may occur, and life may feel unmanageable. Patients may show abnormal tendencies, when people who know them feel they are exhibiting behaviors uncharacteristic to their personality. They should see a doctor immediately and have treatment done before menstruation.

To illustrate the importance of realizing the severity of these symptoms in advance, there are reports showing a high percentage of women that committed suicide or had criminal tendencies undertook these behaviors in the timeframe from four days pre-menstruation to the first four days during menstruation.

In analyzing the case story in this chapter, our patient's change in mood and aggressiveness before menstruating belongs to the second degree of symptoms. This is due to the liver being "on fire." As the primary organ that regulates the movement of qi in the body, this over-abundance can cause a significant change in mood, making one feel aggravated, hot, uneasy and unstable. But why did she also feel tired? This is due to liver fire consuming a lot of energy and disturbing the spleen. When the spleen cannot produce energy and blood, this causes the onset of fatigue. Retention of water is also a symptom of a weakened spleen, showing that it is not able to efficiently transport water throughout the body.

Depression usually happens to women who use birth control pills for many years: pre-menstruation, after child birth and during menopause. Women who use birth control pills more readily show these symptoms of depression, some studies show, because the pills influence hormone levels that have certain links with depression. Usually, if women have a normal balance of sexual hormone levels, then their emotions are more easily harmonized. However, when hormonal levels change, then unbalanced emotion follows.

Another study shows that women with painful menstruation have slower hormonal development, which affects concentration levels and mental capacity at different ages. With heavy bleeding that is prolonged for longer than ten days, women tend to show a stronger dip in emotion, accompanied by heightened activity of the parasympathetic and sympathetic nervous systems, making them feel more symptoms and exacerbating the entire problem.

Bleeding and lack of blood nourishment can also induce mood swings. These mood swings may in turn cause disturbances in the blood vessels and sympathetic nervous system, making them over-active. This creates a counterproductive state, tensing up the body more, further disturbing the blood vessel system and leading to more bleeding—a self-perpetuating cycle.

In many places, there is a cultural belief that these symptoms are inevitable, so this focus may bring them about more strongly. In other words, anticipating the problem may cause or worsen it. For instance, in Asia, post-pregnancy, women tend to be very nervous and cautious to extreme levels (for example, not washing their hair for 30 days or not brushing teeth).

To make a comprehensive conclusion, there are three over-arching factors contributing to emotional changes during menstruation. Firstly, hormonal changes from menstruation cause mood swings and other emotional symptoms by affecting the nervous system. Secondly, women often have a tendency to be influenced strongly by their culture, and their anxiety about the "inevitable" symptoms may exacerbate the problem during this period. Thirdly, one must consider the natural cycle of emotions.

Starting at birth, there is a biological clock that affects physical strength, intelligence and the emotional periodic rhythm of life. This coincides with the natural cycles of days, nights, the sun and the moon. The natural birth cycle of emotions is 28 days and a woman's menstrual cycle is also close to 28 to 30 days.

For example, Ms. Wang was born March 31. Her emotional cycle is as follows: April 3 to 14 being the "high state" of emotion, and April 17 to 28 being the "low state" of emotion. There are about 2 days of transition between each state in which people don't experience either a high or low, feeling stable. During the higher state of emotion, people usually feel happier and have a good attitude towards progress. They deal with things in a more accommodating way and find it easy to forgive and forget. During the lower emotional state, feelings are down and it is easy to worry, be suspicious and see things in a negative light for no reason.

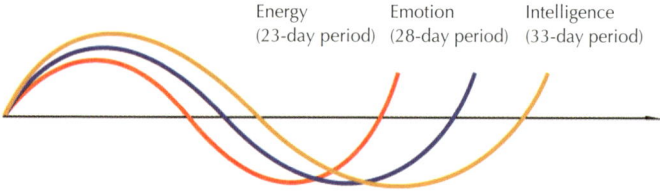

The Natural Cycle of Energy, Emotion and Intelligence

The menstrual hormonal cycle, of course, happens only to women, and therefore, combined with their natural birth cycle of emotion, creates a new overall monthly emotional cycle that we call "The Complex Emotional Cycle."

During 25 years of research and practice, I have recognized two types of emotional states: steady and volatile. If the cycles are closely linked, meaning if the time fourteen days post-menstruation corresponds to the high state of the natural birth cycle of emotion, then the woman tends to have an overall steady emotional state with only mild emotional changes. If this is the opposite, and the emotional birth cycle and hormonal cycle are in conflict or irregular, then the overall emotional state is more violent and volatile.

Continuing to use Ms. Wang as an example, her natural birth emotional cycle is in the high state in the first part of the month and lower in the second half. If her menstruation occurs between the 18th and 25th of the month, then her monthly complex emotional cycle will be more stable. However, if her menstruation arrives between the 3rd and the 10th, her monthly complex emotional cycle will be more violent. And if menstruation occurs between the 11th and 17th or the 26th and the 2nd of the next month, the complex emotional cycle may not be certain, depending on personality, environment, weather, education level and cultural influences to determine its severity.

It is important to acknowledge these two different cycles that affect the overall emotional state during the month. If there are fewer or less severe symptoms, sometimes the emotional state can be managed simply through awareness of stress, maintaining a positive outlook, a nourishing and warm diet, and exercising. For premenstrual tension I have developed certain treatments and recipes to alleviate volatility, putting the body and mind into a more balanced state.

There are two kinds of qi patterns with premenstrual tension. The first is liver qi stagnation in the body, which includes a feeling of depression with mood swings, and tenderness and/or fullness in the breasts. The second is marked by aggressiveness, easily losing temper and migraines—symptoms of excess of yang qi in the liver ("liver fire") that spreads around and out of the body. For the first pattern, it is necessary to open liver meridians to regulate with other meridians. For the second, it is important to counter-flow the meridian qi back to its center.

Therefore, mood is very much a result of stored, stagnated or excessive qi in the body, showing an imbalance of the body and not just the mind. The liver is more responsible for changes in emotion, whereas the heart is more responsible for one's consciousness and spirit. If the liver is able to effectively regulate one's qi and help the blood circulation, it results in a better mood and a higher tolerance for emotional upsets.

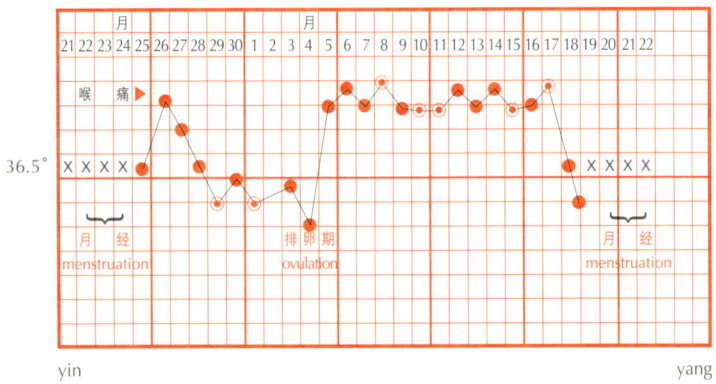

Remedy and Solution

Food options for treating symptoms of mild anger, irritability and aggressiveness

As mentioned above, premenstrual tension commonly has two patterns: One is liver qi stagnation, the other is an upsurge of liver fire. Regulating liver qi, opening energy points and cooling down liver fire can balance excessive anger, tearfulness, irritability, hot temperament and aggressiveness.

Anger with headache, dizziness

Celery. Eat 100g daily as a salad with flavoring of your choice.

Radish 50g, carrot 30g. Eat daily as a salad with flavoring of your choice. Or add 300ml water and cook for 20 minutes and add flavoring for soup.
(Good for hot constitution)

Irritability or tearfulness, depression, or tenderness/fullness of the breasts and hyperchandrake (rib) area

Fresh Chinese hawthorn berry (山楂). Cook 30g with 100ml water and add 5g of honey, drink as decoction. Or use 5g of dry Chinese hawthorn berry to make hot tea, drink 2 cups a day after food.

Dry citrus fruits (柑橘). 5g for hot tea, drink 2 cups a day after food.
(Good for people with qi and blood stagnation)

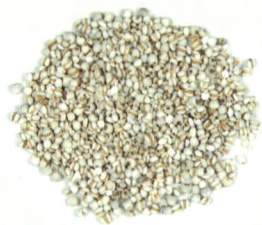

Pearl Barley

Tiger lily buds 黄花菜 (Golden Noodles). Take 50g dried and soak in warm water for 10 minutes, then cut in half. You can mix with any vegetables to stir-fry, or make soup with 1 chicken egg.
(Good for weak and hot constitutions)

Tiger lily buds, also called "forget worry grass" are also good for many conditions e.g. blood-heat type of bleeding, dark-colored bleeding, difficult urination, chest distention, irritability, insomnia, clouded vision and breast infection. Caution: Fresh tiger lily buds can cause food poisoning, only use dried product.

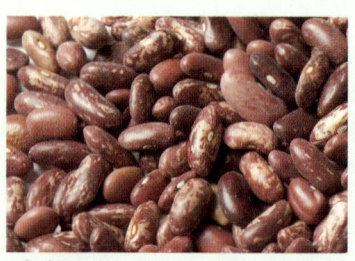

Adzuki Bean

Anger with water retention and fatigue

Pearl barley (Job's tear) 薏苡仁. Cook 30g with 100ml water and add 5g brown sugar. Eat barley and drink soup.

Adzuki bean 赤小豆. Add 30g of the bean to 100g of glutinous rice and mix with 500ml of water to make porridge.
(Good for weak and cold constitutions)

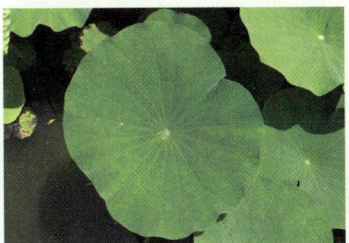
Lotus Leaf

Anger with weight gain and constipation

Cassia seed 决明子. Use 15g of the seed to make tea, 2-3 cups daily.

Lotus leaf powder 荷叶粉. Take 2g daily in capsule.
(Good for hot constitution)

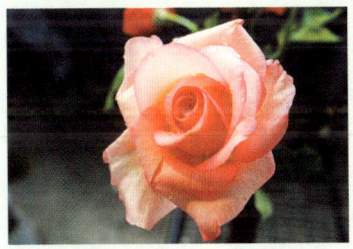
Chinese Rose

Excessive sweet consumption and constant sighing

Cortex Albziae bark or flower 合欢皮或花. Add 10g to 5 Jujubes 红枣 and 150ml water. Cook 15 minutes as decoction, divide in two portions to drink between meals.

Tangerine 橘 and Jujubes 红枣. Eat 2-3 pieces of tangerine or 10 jujubes (dates) when the need for sweet arises.

Chinese Rose flower 月季花. Use 3g to make tea.
(Good for all constitutions)

Cortex Albiziae Bark (*he huan pi* 合欢皮)

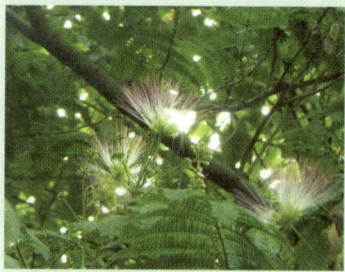

Cortex Albiziae
Photograph by Zhang Yifang

- **Therapeutic Taste and Property:** Sweet, neutral.
- **Function:** Tranquilize the mind and disperse depressed qi, activate blood circulation and relieve swelling.
- **Application:** It is used for emotional injury manifested as mental depression, feeling of restlessness and disquiet, insomnia and amnesia. It is also used for trauma and swelling, as well as for carbuncles and ulcers.
- **Usage and Dosage:** 10-15g is used in decoction for drinking.
- **Note:** The flower or bud of Albiziae Julibrissin Durazz is used as a medicinal herb, named Hehuanhua (Flos Albiziae). It has similar medicinal properties and effects to those of Cortex Albiziae but is especially effective in tranquilizing the mind and dispersing depressed qi, and is usually used for restlessness and disquiet, insomnia, mental depression, amnesia and frequent dreams. Use 6g a day.

Recipe:

Stir-Fried Mushroom with Celery

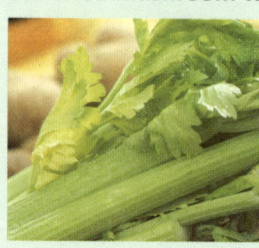

Celery

- **Ingredients:** Celery 400g (chopped), water-soaked straw mushrooms 草菇 50g, salt 3g, 1 teaspoon vinegar, 2 teaspoons dry starch, 1/2 teaspoon soy sauce, olive oil.
- **Preparation:** Put salt, vinegar and starch into a bowl, and add about 50ml of water to make a thin paste. Heat oil in pan, add chopped celery and stir-fry for 2-3 minutes. Add mushrooms, then soy sauce, and after a while add the paste and keep stir-frying quickly.
- **Function:** Treats irritable headache, dizziness caused by upsurge of liver fire.

Self-Acupressure Point

Moving Between (Xingjian 行间)

Location: On the dorsal aspect of the foot, on the web area between the first and second toe, right at the line of changing coloration of skin.

Function: Drains liver fire, cools blood heat, mostly due to subduing rising qi of the liver.

Indication: Irregular or profuse menstruation, insomnia, anger and irritability due to premenstrual tension, epilepsy, convulsions, swelling and painful chest, distension of the abdomen, pain and fullness of the hypochondrium, swelling and pain of the eyes, dizziness and vertigo.

Method: Press counterclockwise for 30 circles, each side of the body separately.

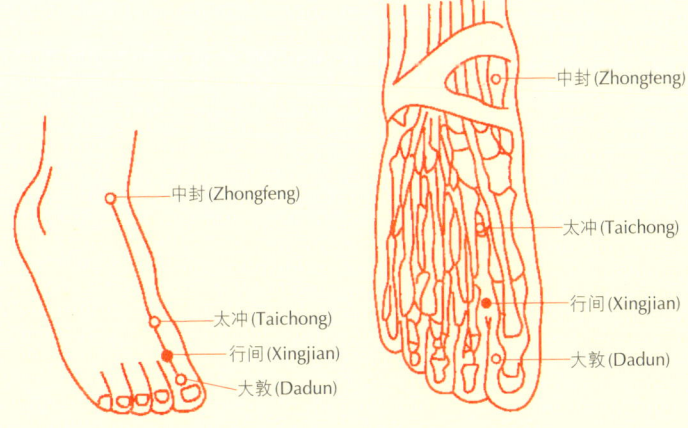

Chapter 5
Managing Emotions throughout Your Life Cycle: the Kidney System

肾者，作强之官，先天之本，主藏精。
——《黄帝内经》

Shen zhe, zuo qiang zhi guan, xian tian zhi ben, zhu cang jing.

The kidney is the administrative organ with the greatest power. The kidney is the congenital base of life and it stores essence

—*Yellow Emperor's Inner Canon*

The kidney acts as the strength and intelligence of the entire body, and is responsible for its overall constitution. It is a storage facility for good essence, and it governs the growth and development of the body as well as the maturation of the reproductive systems. It is the congenital base of life, and while partly based on heritage, one's own health management also influences the kidney's overall state.

TCM divides the transitional life cycle of emotions into ranges. Emotional development from birth to old age is divided as follows: birth to one-year-old, elementary years (ages 1 to 12), pre-teenaged and teenaged years (ages 12 to 20), adult years (ages 20 to 50), retirement years (ages 50 to 60) and elderly years (ages 60+).

There are quick development phases during the period between birth and the age of twenty, when parents need to pay more attention to a child's healthy development. The first phase of development should draw support from both the mother and father. From birth to six-months-old, the child builds up yin energy by spending more time with the mother, through her nurturing. Then, for the rest of the first year, the child is exposed to more yang energy, spending time with the father. This builds up qualities related to yang qi, such as strength, high expectations, tolerance, endurance and bravery. As children grow up, it is important they get the right information from parents and teachers so that they understand their bodies, which leads to a balanced physical and emotional development.

During retirement years, kidney essence is decreased and yin-yang balance levels are downcast, tending more toward fear, and slightly depressed and lonely feelings. The elderly have a tendency then to rely more on their children for attention and for feelings of security and strength. These are all normal feelings and should be expected as a natural way for the body to adapt to physical changes and shifts in qi.

Case Story

A young girl, age ten, began to feel a sudden shift of emotions that would fluctuate between happy and sad. Daydreaming, particularly about boys, became a common way to spend her time. Her daydreaming became excessive and she began, almost involuntarily, to ignore her teachers and parents, becoming tired after snapping back to reality.

The girl's parents took her to the doctor to see if there was anything to be done. She already had her period for one year, starting at the age of nine, and her breasts had slowly developed since the age of eight. Physically, her hormone development started early, but her emotional and mental states were still that of an innocent young girl.

Once her menstrual cycle began, it triggered kidney essence, which produces kidney qi, divided into kidney yin qi or kidney yang qi. Her body responded to this signal to start changing, eventually changing her mood. However, she was not educated about this yet since eleven is the average age to start sex education. Being so young, she was always hiding her early development and storing these emotions, hiding her feelings from her teachers and friends. These complexes then brought about her tendency to daydream and be distant and absent-minded.

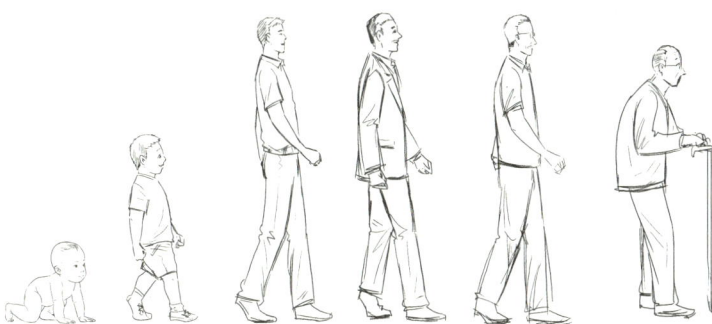

Analysis

According to TCM theory, kidney energy is very important for the growth and development of the mind and the physical body, and especially, the reproductive systems. The Chinese believe in a cycle of seven years for women. At age seven, our baby teeth, hair and body slowly start changing into that of a pre-teen adult. At 14, puberty happens, with highly harmonized kidney energy, and the reproductive system starts to develop, causing menstruation as well as breast and hair growth. After a few years of menstruation, women are able to conceive.

Kidney energy is very important at this time for young girls. Certain kinds of food can hinder or exacerbate kidney energy, and it is possible that the reproductive system can also mature too early. According to recent studies, young girls who have a high consumption of fast food chicken, which is high in hormones, can experience early menstruation and small cysts on the nipples.

At this age, their central nervous systems and brains have not matured to that of a teenager. They can therefore have emotional reactions resulting from this conflict in the body. This condition is called the early maturation of sexual development. If they have a little daydreaming, this is normal during their sexual development, providing a kind of self-release of tension, and it shouldn't be criticized. However, if it is too often and it is affecting their studies and everyday life, then it is important to help harmonize the kidney and heart by using certain foods to help the child relax. However, parents should not be too worried about these symptoms.

After five cycles of seven years (35 years), the surface of the yang meridian starts to decrease, so women start to have wrinkles. After age 42, after six cycles, there is a decrease of kidney energy and reproductive functions also decrease, including changes in menstruation.

After 49, sexual hormones—made by kidney essences—become very low, periods will stop, desire for sex decreases and people cannot get pregnant easily. Some people will have increased menopausal symptoms. Many also experience calcium depletion, having softer or more sensitive teeth, or breaking bones more easily. Hair becomes gray or white and does not grow as thickly as at a younger age. Generally speaking, kidney essence and kidney qi decrease and become unbalanced. This is also demonstrated among menopausal cases by hot flashes, sweating, mood swings, loss in hearing, restless sleep and early waking habits, resulting from disharmony between the kidney and heart.

In TCM, doctors judge kidney essence by examining a patient's teeth, hair, bones and hearing, and by assessing the state of the patient's reproductive system and sexual life. The kidney is the congenital root of healthy development identified through healthy kidney yin and kidney yang. If the kidney qi of both parents is strong and healthy, a child has better chances to be healthy. But it can also be harmonized and regulated through a balanced lifestyle, and the proper food and activities. Even if we cannot change our congenital condition, we can regulate our diet and lifestyle to form the strong kidney foundation needed to maintain a good essence.

In some cases in pre-menopause (average age from 45–55), women may experience symptoms of fear, particularly in front of strangers. They become more distant and uninterested in social events, have a propensity to wake up too early in the morning, experience spotting or missing menstruations four to five times a year. After menstruation is finished, migraines are common with pressure on the eyes, an inability to focus and, sometimes, nausea, vomiting and noises in the ear. The tongue is usually pale and pulses are deeper and weaker.

Men also have a form of menopause but it is not as commonly apparent as in women. The usual age range is 55 to 65. Men experiencing this condition tend to be more violent and feel muscle discomfort or headaches despite normal results from medical examinations. They may feel less focused and motivated, as well as having an overall apprehension about how to conduct themselves.

Advice for men going through this is similar to that of women going through menopause: Tonify the kidney to harmonize with the liver and heart and achieve a better balance. Swimming is strongly encouraged to help the yang energy open up to prevent stagnation. In general, finding hobbies to stay distracted and productive is the best way to alleviate these problems.

It is important to note that this is not an illness that needs to be resolved but is a natural part of the life cycle. In Western medicine, there is a belief that our metabolism slows down and there is decreased coordination between the immune, nervous and hormone systems. In Chinese medicine, the belief is that the kidney essence has decreased and is no longer in harmony with other major *zang-fu* organs, particularly the heart and liver. Therefore, all treatment concentrates on bringing better harmony between these organs. The first advice is to make a change in lifestyle, insisting on regular sleep, exercise, regulated eating patterns, always eating breakfast and drinking lots of water. Taking more vegetables and fruits high in vitamin B is also advantageous.

Since kidney function plays such an important role, it

is vital to understand how the emotions affect the kidneys. Out of the seven emotions, fear most easily disturbs the kidney's function. In the early times, fear had the benefit of keeping humans away from danger and aware of dangerous situations. Research shows that when we are afraid, most of our energy and blood circulates to the big joints and muscles, and all attention is put into making the decision to get out of the situation. This is part of the reaction of the body during this time.

Fear continues to plays an important role in the development of an individual's life cycle of emotions. Anxiety and nervousness are a mild degree of fear. As described previously, before important examinations, students often get extremely anxious and nervous, but this can be good, causing increased awareness and blood flow. However, if anxiety is too prolonged, it will bring negative results, especially when it develops into fear, which disturbs kidney energy.

There are two types of fear in TCM: One is situational and one is self-produced. Being frightened by a situation is brought on by external circumstances and causes kidney qi to be deficient and flow downward, but also disperses or causes imbalance of heart qi. Fear that is self-produced, considered to be more "worry," holds kidney qi inside the body. Though the symptoms may look the same, understanding the cause or root of the fear is important for the diagnosis and treatment. For fear that affects the heart, it is common for patients to have insomnia and reverberated effects of imbalances from this fear (i.e. nightmares and restless sleep). They need to be treated immediately to help harmonize heart and kidney systems. For self-inflicted fear, a good way to control it is to stay busy, allowing the patient to be distracted. (More on fear can be found in Chapter 1.)

Remedy and Solution

Food options for treating symptoms caused by the transitions of puberty and menopause

1. Food options for children going through puberty

Children from all nations are more commonly experiencing earlier sexual development due to poor diet, environmental changes and over-exposure to adult content through media. TCM believes this condition is due to having a hot constitution.

Difficulty concentrating

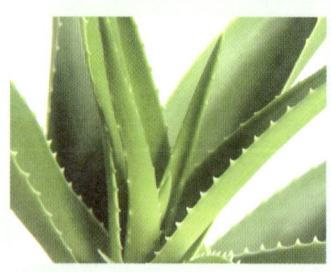
Aloe vera

Lingzhi mushrooms 灵芝. Take 2 capsules a day or 1g of extract powder, 6g of dry herb.
(Good for all constitutions) (See also chapter 7)

Chrysanthemum flower 菊花 3g.

Aloe vera 芦荟. Take 100ml juice or yogurt daily before food.
(Good for hot constitution) (See also chapter 2)

For children with difficulty concentrating, constipation

Jujube (Chinese red date) 红枣 and black fungus 黑木耳. Take 20 jujubes and 6 pieces of fungus, and make tea. Children under 2 years old should have for 2 days.
(Good for blood and yin weakness in any season)

Boat-fruited sterculia seed 胖大海. Use one piece to make a tea, and add 2 teaspoons to juice, 2 times a day.
(Good for hot constitution)

2. Food options for menopause

The emotional disturbances of menopause are various: Some people get easily fretful, agitated, angry, annoyed and worried, while some feel unhappy with a propensity to cry, and often feel out of control. Different people have different reactions, such as the duration of an emotion or mood swing and the category of symptoms. The influenced meridian and *zang-fu* organs also differ due to the decreasing kidney qi and the individual's particular constitution, profession, diet and overall lifestyle.

The imbalance of the kidney will bring disorder to other systems. Dialectical treatment, which addresses the balance between or regulates systems, will be used with the kidney as the root of the issue. The treatment is based on the emotion displayed as a reaction to the imbalance. For instance, if someone is easily agitated and angered, the treatment will focus on coordinating the liver and kidney. If someone feels worried and sad, one must coordinate the kidney and lung. If someone is over-thinking, vexed and suffering from insomnia, one must coordinate the heart, spleen and kidney systems. Therefore, emotion during menopause is a complex reaction to an imbalance of the organs and meridian systems, and needs to be treated accordingly.

For women

Hot flashes, mood swings and hyperawareness of the body

Lotus plumule 莲心. Use 2g, add 100ml of boiling water. Leave lid on for 10 minutes, then drink while warm.

Bamboo leaf 淡竹叶 and Artemisia annua berb 青蒿. Add 10g of each to 600 ml water to decoct. Divide into two portions to drink.
(Good for hot constitution)

Immature wheat grain 浮小麦 30g, licorice 甘草 6g, 10 pieces of jujubes 红枣 (Chinese red date), 5 pieces of dry longan 桂圆. Mix with water to make a soup.
(Good for nervous sweat, mood swings and hyperawareness of the body with all constitutions. You should also reduce spices, limit wine drinking and smoking to have a better response.)

(For more sleeplessness and palpitation remedies, see chapter 2)

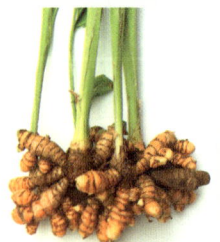
Turmeric Rhizome

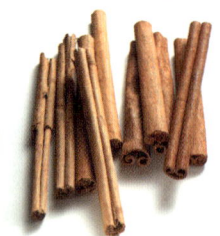
Cinnamon

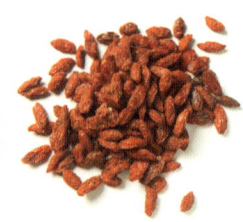
Wolfberry

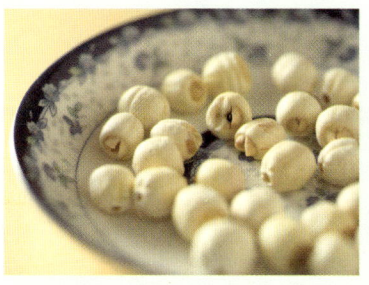
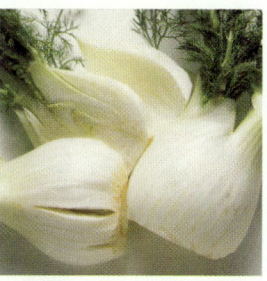

Lotus Seed (with Plumule Inside)   Fennel

For men

Sense of fear, hopelessness or non-productivity

Slightly spicy food, e.g. cinnamon 肉桂 3g or fennel 小茴香 6g. Take daily with food.
(Good for cold and weak constitutions)

Turmeric rhizome 姜黄. Use 10g for tea.
(Good for stagnation of qi and blood)

Chinese leek seed 韭菜子 10g and Chinese raspberry 覆盆子 10g for decoction. Or wolfberry 枸杞子 10g and schisandra berry 五味子 10g for decoction.
(Good for kidney qi and yin weakness)

Anger and high blood pressure, high cholesterol and a fatty liver

Lily bulb 百合. Stir-fry 50g with 150g of celery daily.
Cassia seed 决明子. Use 15g for 2 cups of tea.
(Good for hot constitution)

Hawthorn berry 10g. Steam with 5 pieces of jujube (Chinese red date) for 10 minutes, then eat.
(Good for cold constitution)

Semen Biota Seed (*bai zi ren* 柏子仁)

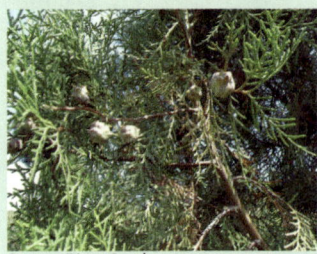

Semen Biota Seed
Photograph Courtesy of Herbasinica, Shenyang, China

- **Therapeutic Taste and Property:** Sweet, neutral.
- **Function:** Nourish the heart and tranquilize the mind, moisten the intestines and relax the bowels. Good for any kind of constitution.
- **Application:** It is indicated for deficiency of heart qi or insufficiency of heart yin, and failure of the heart to be nourished, manifested as vexation, insomnia, convulsions and epilepsy.

It is used for constipation due to dryness of the intestine, especially for that due to yin deficiency and insufficiency of the blood since Semen Biota Seed is moistening and excessively oily in property.

- **Usage and Dosage:** 3-9g is used in decoction for drinking.
- **Note:** It is used with caution in cases with loose stool and excessive sputum.

Recipe:

Lotus Seed and Lily Bulb Congee

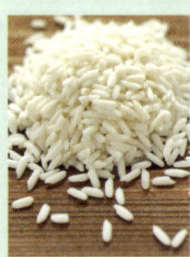

Glutinous Rice

- **Ingredients:** Lotus seed 莲子 30g, lily bulb 百合 50g, wolfberry 枸杞 10g, glutinous rice 糯米 50g.
- **Preparation:** Soak ingredients for 20 minutes. Put rice, lotus seed and lily bulb into earthenware pot and add water. After water comes to a boil, reduce heat and stew for 30 minutes, then add wolfberry for 2 minutes. Sweeten with honey. Eat once in the morning, once at night.
- **Function:** Relieves palpitations, sleeplessness, poor memory, fatigue. Good for tonifying kidney yin and reducing heart fire to harmonize kidney and heart.

Date and White Fungus Custard

• **Ingredients:** White fungus 银耳 10g and wolfberry 枸杞 10g, 6 pieces of jujubes (Chinese red date) 红枣, corn 玉米 20g and Chinese yam powder 山药粉 20g.

• **Preparation:** Soak white fungus for half an hour, and then wash jujubes and wolfberry and corn. Cook white fungus and jujubes until they become soft then add wolfberry, corn and Chinese yam and stir well. Add crystal sugar or honey to serve.

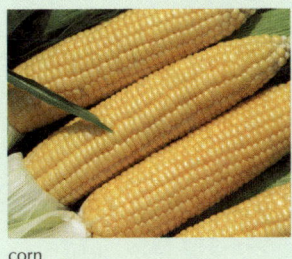
corn

• **Function:** Tonifys yin and blood, nourishes and removes dryness, calms the mind. Treats weak body constitution and ensures deep sleep.

(There are other herbal pills that may suit specific menopausal symptoms—please consult with your TCM doctor.)

Self-Acupressure Point

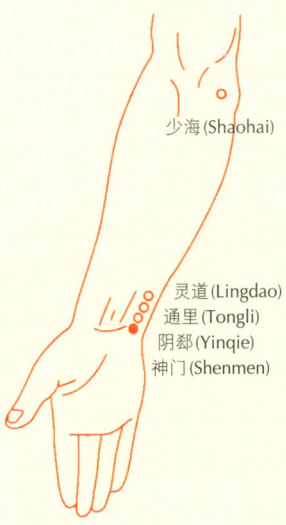

Spirit Gate (Shenmen 神门)

Location: Between the first and second wrist crease, in the depression on the little finger side of your inner arm.

Function: Quiets the heart and spirit, clears fire and cools hot constitution, clears heart heat, regulates qi counter flow.

Indication: Cardiac pain, irritability, palpitations, hysteria, amnesia, insomnia, mania and epilepsy. Also helps balance menopausal symptoms.

Method: Use fingernail or tip to press the point in counterclockwise and clockwise circles, 20 times respectively.

Chapter 6
Managing Emotions according to Gender: the Digestive System (Spleen)

脾胃者，仓廪之官，五味出焉，后天之本。
——《黄帝内经》

*Pi wei zhe, cang lin zhi guan,
wu wei chu yan, hou tian zhi ben.*

The spleen and stomach organs transport and store food and nutrition, and are responsible for digestion, absorption and the transmission of flavors. The spleen and stomach form the postnatal base of life.

—*Yellow Emperor's Inner Canon*

In TCM, the spleen and stomach make up the entire digestive system, and include the pancreas, small intestine and part of the stomach functions as they are known in Western medicine. The spleen is the "Agricultural Bureau" of the body, controlling where energy "seeds" are planted and how the health of the body is harvested. The spleen is the post-natal base of life, meaning once all the congenital factors of the body have been determined, one's health management relies on the spleen to do the rest of the work.

阴阳异质，男女殊料。

——万全

Yin yang yi zhi, nan nü shu liao.

The properties of yin and yang are different; the material bases of male and female are different.

—Wan Quan

Males build up more yang, showing tall, strong and stable-bodied characteristics. Females build up more yin, so that their outward image is slender, soft and flexible. Therefore, due to the difference in yin and yang, men and women have many differences in their physiological functions and psychological state, and their coping abilities are different as well. As a broad generalization, men are partial to physical strength and women are partial to emotion. Yin and yang are complementary essences, as are the male and female essences, and men and women can often reinforce each other's qi when they live together.

Case Story 1

Mr. Wen, managing director of an advertising company, decided at the age of 40 to condense his planned career and take an early retirement, ten years short of the average retirement age, in order to enjoy freedom and relaxation at an earlier age. Therefore, he worked extremely hard. From Monday to Friday, he left home early and returned late, work overtime for a total of 12 to 15 hours daily. On weekends, other than two hours of exercise, he continued working, either at home or in the office, with only the occasional Sunday off.

During any free time, he would take on additional MBA studies—increasing his mental and physical stress. In the past three years, Mr. Wen's highly specialized management expertise had brought the attention of many recruitment agencies, who would call him constantly, seeing whether he wanted to change companies. His personal goal was to eventually become the CEO of an international company. In two years time, he had changed his company twice, adding even more pressure with each change, as he had to adapt to a different working culture, with new employees and new company goals.

He decreased his sleeping hours to make more time for work and study, sometimes waking up in the middle of the night dreaming or sleep-talking about his experiences during the day. Waking the following day, he felt drained, and had to rely on six or seven cups of coffee to keep himself awake.

After continuing like this for over a year, his nervous system was distraught, and his neck muscles became tight. He began experiencing irritable bowel syndrome with early morning abdominal pain and soft stool. After two more weeks, all the muscles in his shoulder and upper back became very tight and sore, and his neck became extremely stiff. An onset of dizzy spells with nausea caused him to worry and he rushed to the hospital for a check-up. The doctor checked his body and couldn't find anything wrong, except for the irritable bowel syndrome and stress-related anxiety.

At this point, Mr. Wen decided to stop and re-evaluate the physical symptoms that were being caused by his lifestyle habits. His passion and energy for his job—something he used to always have—had decreased recently. His body energy could no longer cope, and at work, he could no longer be the person he used to be under these circumstances. Doubts of ever being able to handle his dream job of CEO began to take over his thoughts, dampening his confidence and making him re-evaluate his position and career goals. His strong will and confidence had been transformed because of his physical state. This is a case of over-thinking, over-planning and exhausting one's mental state combined with physical exhaustion, leading to fatigue.

Case Story 2

Ms. Rui worked for an IT company as a program manager. After the delivery of her daughter, she had post-natal depression. She started to experience lower back soreness and heel pain after returning to her daily chores. Although she thought she was having enough rest and good food, these two symptoms did not subside after two weeks. Then she started to feel very sad and depressed. Even when she saw the happy smile of her daughter, she could not be joyful, and was often tearful and quiet around the home. Her parents worried that she was unhappy to deliver a daughter though this was not at all the case.

Before Ms. Rui had the child, she had a very important position in the company and was due for a promotion, and when she became pregnant, it postponed her career. She was determined to go back to work two months after having her baby. Within the first month, she became apprehensive that she would be unable to become healthy enough to return to work, and that delaying her return would mean that her promotion would go to someone else. Therefore, she cried several times without letting her parents see, and eventually even got eye pain.

Her demeanor became very worrisome and small issues became big deals. She fell into a depressed state, thinking that this child had disturbed her physical condition and career aspirations, associating the child with her apparent shortcomings and weakened physical state. Clinically, we also see many women getting depressed easily after their second child, as the women's parents and relatives may not be as involved as they were for the first-born.

Analysis

In TCM, "over-thinking" belongs to one of the seven emotions. The original meaning of "over-thinking" in the Chinese context has two origins. This first is during puberty when raging hormones cause teenagers to start having emotional changes. They have feelings towards the opposite sex, but repress them, turning the feelings into a type of longing or desire that is not fully understood or manifested. Some are open to talking about it with friends or family, while some keep it suppressed and it becomes a bottled-up type of longing. This is never treated in Western medicine, which considers it a natural phase of development. In TCM, this is a very real phenomenon that can go overboard, particularly in societies, like that in parts of China, where there is no culture of speaking openly about this emotion. For example, there have been cases of pop idolization where crazed fans actually believe they have truly fallen in love with a star, sometimes even going to the lengths of committing suicide or becoming physically ill because of these emotions.

The second origin comes from pondering one's future, career and personal goals. A passion for work is natural and healthy, as are self-reflection and an interest in personal progress by making well-evaluated choices. But many times, it becomes an obsession. If this over-thinking starts to disturb sleep, eating habits and bowel movements, then one's body has already given signals that the over-thinking has become stressful and unmanageable.

Over-thinking in TCM disturbs the heart and spleen systems: The heart starts to pump faster, causing the spleen and stomach to respond with quicker movements and the production of more acid, and energy flows downwards. Over-thinking can block the energy of other organs because all the qi and blood is in the brain, causing other organs to be energy-deficient, and therefore move or respond more slowly. Reduced hunger and picky eating, muddy thinking and fatigue are often symptoms of this stagnation. Both of them will disturb the digestive system; if there is disharmony between liver and spleen, stress-related abdominal pain and diarrhea occurs.

Emotion can affect the spleen and liver, and disharmony between these two essential organs can also cause certain emotions. Sometimes when an organ is of excess heat constitution, for instance the liver, the result can be a bad temperament or aggressiveness. Or, if the spleen energy is deficient, people can lack energy and the ability to plan for the future and not have good sleep.

In TCM, the spleen is not just a digestive organ but also the root of acquired constitution. It is the source of energy and blood for the entire bodily system. If these symptoms last for a longer time, there can be a genuine deficiency of energy and blood, causing fatigue and exhaustion. The spleen is also responsible for willpower, clear thinking and confidence. Chinese parents often look at their child's eating habits to understand the child's level of willpower. Overeating or not eating the right things indicates a lack of willpower, and children who are better at rationing, understanding what is good for them and not over-indulging in sweets are those who have, overall, more control and confidence.

In severe cases, over-thinking can cause depression. My father and grandfather solved more than ten cases of this type. One of my father's patients, Mr. Li, over-used his brain and had emotional disharmony from his relationship. He eventually experienced symptoms like insomnia, dizziness and light-headedness during the day. He became very worried and suspicious; he was often sad and sporadically cried. Many times he would talk to himself. He lost his appetite completely and was constantly thirsty. He always felt like something was stuck in his throat but was unable to clear it.

The hospital psychology department diagnosed him with depression. After using herbal treatments for two weeks, his sleep became much better and his emotional state slightly changed. After two months of treatment, he returned to normal.

Clinical studies and research papers in China show men are more easily disturbed by over-thinking, eventually leading to aggression or bad temper. One likely reason could be that in ancient times, men were often sent out to face the dangers of the wild, whereas women stayed at home or with the clan. Evolutionarily, men were the stronger species in the wild, surviving the elements and standing guard against other species. Men have a higher ability to instinctually smell out danger and react quickly to a scenario. This created the male instinct to try to dominate and aggressively pursue goals.

In modern society, this instinctual behavior is found in career drive and athletic ability. Therefore, males often demonstrate stronger career aspirations and increased competitive behavior in athletics. There are cases of male athletes with tough minds and bodies (even gold medalists) using steroids or consuming a large amount of red meat to increase their natural ability to improve or succeed. Through constant usage, their bodies become too "yang," which in turn, consumes body yin energy. Eventually, it is easy to lose one's temper, become aggressive, emotional or fight easily. Some men may ultimately experience heart disease or failure. There are some stories of athletes dying in the stadium from an extreme imbalance of yin-yang, even in their twenties.

Women must be conscious of tendencies specific to their gender as well. According to Chinese medicine, post-natal emotional disturbance usually falls into three categories: The first is fear during labor, when a woman has unexpected pain and the trauma of her first delivery.

The second is post-delivery, where she feels very weak and tired. Chinese believe that before labor, the pregnant woman is like a "big hot ball of energy" and post-delivery becomes a "small ball of ice"—illustrating the need for extreme care and attention. If the mother meets with unexpected results (like a complication during delivery, a problem with the health of the child, or disappointment about the child's sex), she may have a tendency to let the fear take over and fall into post-natal depression, unable to accept the situation.

The third is a prolonged case of the vagina not closing within the first two weeks post-delivery, with continuous discharge. This makes the woman weaker, and simultaneously, easily susceptible to the environment, catching diseases. In this weakened state, the extraneous invasions of viral or bacterial influences mix with the discharge, building up excess heat, burning up good energy and creating blood deficiency—all of which has a large effect on the mood.

For new mothers who have no energy, feel tearful and experience sadness and unrest on a continuous basis, it is important to have an evaluation. Periods of crying and feeling low are normal in most circumstances, but close monitoring of the first few weeks after delivery is necessary to make sure it is not continuous, which can have consequences on a woman's health. Should the woman fall under any viral or bacterial infection, she should see a doctor immediately.

According to TCM, after child-birth, the energy, blood and kidney essence qi are much weaker than usual. Ms. Rui's case exemplifies this. At that same time, the body has to face a new change; during pregnancy, the body is going through a state of "storage," when menstruation stops and the body focuses on nourishing itself to support the child. Once the child is delivered, the body goes through various forms of "release": discharge, breast milk, some tears and sweat. These are a natural bodily reaction to creating a balance between various systems: the kidney and the liver (tears and recovery of the uterus), the liver and stomach (for the breast milk), and the kidney and lung (for the skin and the hair). Some women will also have sloughing of the skin or hair falling out—this is also a type of natural release and regeneration of the body.

It is important to have some of these reactions in order to simulate the natural change within the body. This is a unique time in a woman's development. One must use special care with food within the first ten days—particularly with warm foods or drinks to protect the uterus. Secondly, foods that regulate blood (such as red bean soup, longan soup or herb jelly) are very important to rebuild strength and encourage the uterus to shrink back to its normal size. After ten days, women can take heavier "tonic" foods, which contain oil, meat and fish.

If there are any unexpected emotional symptoms, these can be tonified through the organ system. Tearfulness and unexpected anger can be handled by solving kidney weakness and liver stagnation. Ms. Rui had three weeks of acupuncture, twice a week, combined with Chinese herbal medicine. She recovered and went back to work after three months.

The location of the deficiency or stagnation also has to do with people's original constitution—a person's excess liver heat may cause a weak kidney system condition or affect lung yin; long-term weakness of the lung may lead to spleen or kidney qi deficiency. As you can see, one constitutionally-deficient system can affect another, and

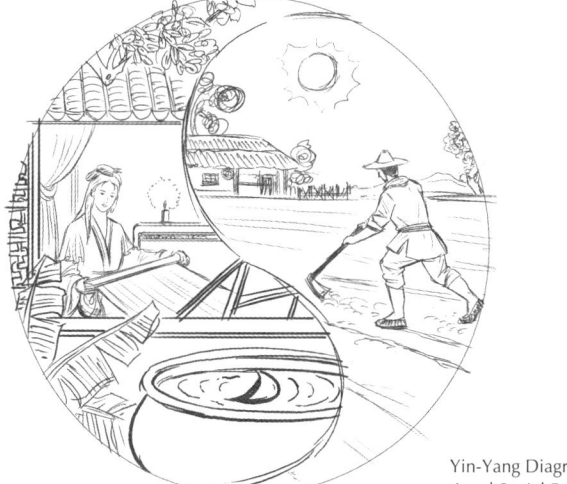

Yin-Yang Diagram Indicating the Traditional Social Role of Man and Woman

in turn, that may eventually weaken the original system. Therefore, it is paramount for people to lead balanced lives to improve their original physical constitution. (Please also refer to chapter 3 and chapter 4 for more information on sadness and on anger and aggressiveness as related to the complex emotional cycle.)

In general, TCM believes that compared with men, women's constitution and overall temperament belong to the yin energy, with a soft, flexible, "watery" physical and emotional state. Society treats men and women differently, believing they have different characters and roles. Female intuition and understanding is rooted in a general tendency to respect and care for others, especially men and parents. Most women are more concerned about emotional matters, and can also experience very detailed emotions compared to men. They tend to be more sensitive to external emotions and usually have more extreme emotional ups-and-downs.

Research shows that anxiety and depression may happen more often in women than men, while men are more easily affected by over-thinking and aggressiveness. One famous

TCM doctor's case study research showed that physical changes were caused by emotions in only 5.5% of men, but for women, it was 15.2%. Anxiety and worry occurs six times more in women than men; this is why sadness and worry are considered "of female property or essence."

As stated previously, the male principle is related to yang energy; more aggressive and able to argue, men are biologically built to release emotion through confrontation. During social activities, men are more prone to smoking and drinking wine and coffee, and they also often exhibit work stress. But according to TCM, these are highly "yang" oriented, making them even more "yang."

Clinically, research shows that instead of being caused by organ imbalance, high blood pressure is an original state that leads to organ imbalance, brought on by external influences and building up yang qi on an already yang body. When meeting the same circumstance, men and women usually react in very different ways: Women may be faced with indecision and anxiety, whereas men want to take action, solve the problem or fight. In TCM, we usually believe women have more repressed liver qi and men have counter-rising liver qi, both imbalanced states having opposite effects.

From either the Eastern or Western societal perspective, there is a general consensus that men tend to be more competitive and aggressive, forgetful and tolerant, whereas women are softer, gentler and quieter. In today's society, many career women are in the same positions of authority as men but are expected to go home and be gentle, loving and attentive housewives and mothers. The conflict of expectations leads to even greater emotional imbalance and can create feelings of guilt, remorse and questioning one's identity as a woman.

The famous Chinese philosopher Yan Yonghe said, "To treat women's problems caused by emotions will be ten times more difficult than to treat men." A famous anthropologist, Ashley Montagu, believed women were biologically stronger than men. For example, they have a higher pain threshold, which allows them to bear childbirth, and during threatening life situations, their willpower and endurance is much stronger than a man's. In extreme cases of abandonment (for example, if a girl is orphaned), the female constitution is often much stronger than the male, via endurance through immunity and bodily strength.

Women should be aware that they are able to go through large ranges of emotional strife but have the biological makeup to overcome these challenges through the strength of their bodily support system. Understanding that emotion should not control you is an important awareness during a moment of panic and sadness. You can do something to address the stagnations and handle the emotions. Many women, after several failures or catastrophes, have a tendency to give up. But knowing that the female physical body has the ability to "open another kitchen" or overcome these circumstances, as long as the mind stays open, is important to remember.

It is vital to identify the trigger and ascertain the severity of the unhappiness or depression. Unhappiness commonly lasts a short time; overall, the day or week is enjoyable. Depression that lasts more than a few days needs extra attention. A change in attitude—finding a way to help others or trying to find the positive side of things—can already remedy the situation.

Open the curtains and door, share feelings with friends or write them down. Do not lock yourself indoors and, especially, be sure to get out of bed and not sleep too much.

Remedy and Solution

Food options for treating symptoms of mild "over-thinking," longing and pensiveness

Over-thinking, longing and pensiveness easily causes spleen (digestive system) qi stagnation, so we need to promote stomach movement and open the blockage, smooth the qi and loosen the mind. Long-term over-thinking can also cause disharmonious spleen and heart systems, decreasing the quantity and quality of the heart's blood, and at the same time, inducing spleen qi weakness. We advise you to have a broad and balanced diet, take foods that are easy to digest, and tailor your diet to suit your individual body constitution.

Poor appetite, bloated abdomen and stomach, gassiness

Raw Garlic. Eat 1 slice, then take 50ml of warm water.

Clove 丁香. Use 3g as flavoring for salad or soup.

Jasmine flower 茉莉花 tea and barley sprout 麦芽 tea.
(Good for cold and weak constitutions)

Radish. Eat 50g raw. Or make soup with other vegetables, eat 200ml daily. There is an old Chinese saying, "if there is a radish in the kitchen, the pharmacy will close down." That means the radish is a very powerful functional food, particularly for cooling down, detoxifing and soothing the digestive system.

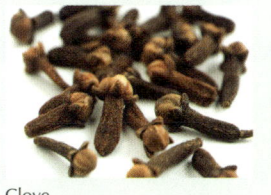
Clove

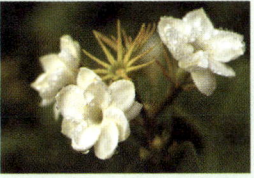
Jasmine

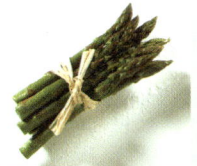
Asparagus

Asparagus. Steam 50g with 2 slices of garlic for 5 minutes.
(Good for hot and week constitutions)

Feelings of a heavy body or muddy head, fatigue

"Same-year" Green tea. Use 5g for tea, drink 2-3 cups daily.

Evergreen tea 苦丁茶. Use 2g, drink 2-3 cups daily.

Lemon juice. One cup a day for 3 days.

Chinese cabbage. Stir-fry 50g or make soup.
(Good for hot constitution and in summer)

Cabbage. Stir-fry 50g with 30g of pepper, take 2 times daily.

Soy bean milk. Drink 100ml warm on an empty stomach.
(Good for cold constitution or in winter)

Anxiety, insomnia, forgetfulness, poor appetite, soft stools

Pearl powder 珍珠粉. Take 2g with warm water 30 minutes before sleep.
(Good for hot constitution and in summer)

Semen Euryales (*qian shi* 芡实)

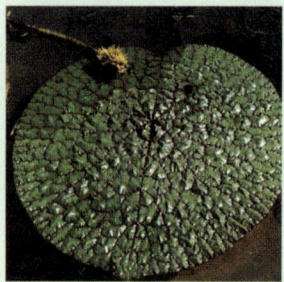

Semen Euryale

• **Therapeutic Taste and Property:** Sweet, neutral, astringent.
• **Function:** Stabilizes the will and calms spirit-mind, strengthens the kidney and astringent essence, firms the spleen and stops diarrhea.
• **Application:** Treats emission, leucorrhea (vaginal discharge), frequent urine and diarrhea.
• **Usage and Dosage:** 15-20g is used in decoction or powder for eating.
• **Contraindication:** Constipation or obstructed urine, indigestion.

Recipe:

Gui Pi Decoction

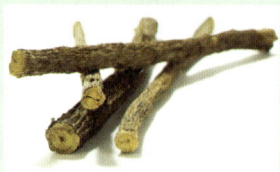

Licorice

• **Ingredients:** Longan 桂圆 30g, licorice 甘草 10g, 10 jujubes 红枣 (Chinese red date), Semen Ziziphus spinosa 酸枣仁 10g, polygala root 远志 10g.
• **Preparation:** Add water (to a level of 3cm over dry ingredients) and soak for 30 minutes. Bring to a boil then simmer for 30 minutes. Pour off and reserve liquid. Add water and boil again, adding this to the first batch of liquid. Stir, and drink half in the morning and half in the evening.
• **Function:** Tonifies spleen qi and heart blood, treats deficiencies due to over-thinking, poor appetite, soft stools, mild irritability, anxiety, insomnia, forgetful, heavy dreaming, pale face, scanty menstruation and palpitations.

Chinese Angelica Root and Mutton Soup (*dang gui yang rou geng*)

• **Ingredients:** Chinese angelica root 当归 (Radix Angelicae Sinensis) 15g, Astragalus root (Radix Astragali seu Hedysari) 黄芪 25g, mutton 500g, 2 spring

onions, 5 pieces of fresh ginger, 1 teaspoon cooking wine and salt 5g.
- **Preparation:** Wash the mutton. Put Chinese Angelica roots and astragalus roots into a gauze bag and tie, put with other ingredients into an earthenware pot. Add water to a level of 5cm over ingredients. Bring to a boil, then stew until the mutton is thoroughly done, about an hour.
- **Direction:** Eat the mutton and drink the soup, twice a day, in the morning and in the evening.
- **Function:** Tonify energy and nourish the blood after illness or delivery. Treat symptoms manifested as depression or postnatal depression, abdominal cold-pain, cold sensation in uterus, prolonged vagina discharge and other kinds of anemia.
- **Contraindication:** Those who have a fever due to infection, painful swelling in the throat and toothache should not eat such soup. Do not use copperware or eat pumpkin.

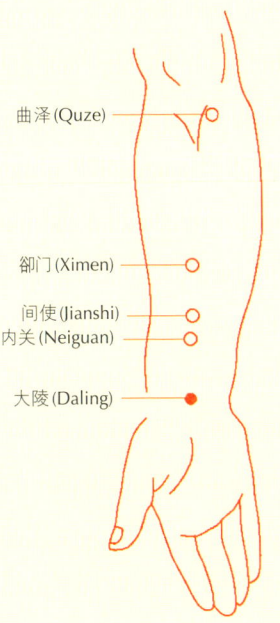

Self-Acupressure Point

Great Mound (Daling 大陵)

Location: At the midpoint of the inner wrist crease, between the two major tendons of the wrist.

Function: Clears the heart and quiets the spirit, harmonizes the stomach and loosens the chest, cools the hot constitution and the blood.

Indication: Treats heart pain and palpitation, stomach pain, palpitations due to fright, mania and withdrawal, mental disorders, epilepsy, stuffy chest, pain in the hypochondriac region (the upper, lateral abdominal region just below the ribs), insomnia, irritability, foul breath.

Method: Use fingernail or ball pen to press the point up and down.

Chapter 7
Managing Emotions according to the Seasons

人与天地相参也，与日月相应也。
——《黄帝内经》

Ren yu tian di xiang can ye, yu ri yue xiang ying ye.

The functions of the human body depend on the Tianqi (Heaven-Qi) and Diqi (Earth-Qi), and adjust in accordance with the movements of the sun and the moon.

—*Yellow Emperor's Inner Canon*

The human body always needs to adapt to and coordinate with the Earth and its seasons. There is a very important relationship between human beings and the Earth. Our physiological functions and emotions and our ability to recover also follow the changes in nature. For instance, our internal organs, meridians, energy and blood movements as well as our emotional cycle are all influenced by the four seasons. TCM uses the rules of nature to help guide people's healthcare and prevent certain illnesses.

Case Story

Ms. Yang, a 39-year-old research staff member at a university, was well-advanced in her academic career. She managed several projects for the Central Government and she was well-regarded by the academic community. However, she had her own angst, often unbeknownst to others. Every winter, there would come a time where her emotions would dip, causing her to be constantly tearful and sad. She felt anxiety and distress, and while most people sleep more heavily in the winter, her sleep was light and disturbed. Sometimes she ate excessively as well. For the past three winters, these symptoms were noticeable. When added with her period, she found her emotions to be particularly different; she did not want to be social or meet new people, her chest and upper abdomen felt tight and sometimes she even felt that life had no meaning.

Analysis

Research in chronobiology, a field of science that examines periodic (cyclic) phenomena in living organisms, states that a human being's physiology and emotions have a strong link with seasonal changes. Chronobiology specific to TCM is based on a holistic view of factors: the environment, season, time of day, person's age, and harmony among organs and qi flow. This differs from the Western theory, which focuses on different gland functions and specific locales in the body.

People often say they have Seasonal Affective Disorder (S.A.D). There are three different reasons:

1) The colder weather of autumn and winter lowers metabolism and there is a decrease of physical functions. This causes slower blood circulation, and the energy support to the brain and sympathetic and parasympathetic nervous systems is more sluggish.

2) There is a gland in the central nervous system of the brain, the conarium, which releases melatonin. Lack of sunlight will increase the gland's production while decreasing adrenal and thyroid hormone production. Once there is a deficiency of these hormones in the blood, the cells and tissues will lack activity, and therefore people feel depressed, fatigued and in a low mood. Sunlight therapy can inhibit over-production of melatonin.

3) *"Jing se xiao se"*: Bleak scenery, lifeless nature and the image of a black crow is often the portrait of autumn/winter, an environment that conjures old memories and provides a slow time of reflection, making us more sad. If there is something that causes irritation, angst or sadness, the autumn and winter seasons usually produce a stronger emotion, linking the seasons with changes in emotional degrees.

In Western psychology, there is a point system that ranks the relative severity of life situations that affect the emotions. For instance, the loss of a partner is the most emotionally distressing situation, with 110 points, while the loss of a child is ranked at 102 and the loss of parents at 96. This point system takes into effect various factors, such as age and length of time one has been involved in this situation, but it misses the seasonal factor. This is another example of how TCM enhances different psychological theories.

In TCM theory, spring and summer are yang seasons,

autumn and winter are yin seasons. All yin-yang energy is influenced by the flow and ebb of seasons. Energy grows in the spring (*chun sheng*), reaching the highest level of the year in summer (*xia zhang*). Energy holds back in the autumn (*qiu shou*), and goes into quiet storage in the winter (*dong cang*).

In the spring, people's emotions mimic the regeneration of other species like plants, or animals after a winter's hibernation. Upon waking, their vitality is restored to a full level. Human emotion can vary widely, as this quick jump into spring can induce many changes, such as feeling sleeping in daytime, hay fever, facial skin rashes, and, especially, an increase in sexual drive. It can also bring on recurred psychoses in the extreme. The body tends to go through a time when rising energy levels need to be channeled. An inability to release sexual drive during this time causes emotional disorders and imbalances in the body.

Summer is a time of rising heat, so people sweat a lot, metabolism increases and emotions are more yang and more outwardly expressive. It's the time of the year when people are more extroverted and generally more happy and enthused. However, if people do not sleep enough and the weather is more humid, then "heat or damp" people have a tendency to feel more annoyed and agitated. If people in the "heat" constitution like to eat red meat, they could become more irritable and angry as they have too much yang.

In early autumn, the weather goes back to the cooling state, the atmosphere becomes more dry and leaves change color. It is usually a very soothing, enjoyable and relaxing time of the year. However, as the season progresses, the cooling air turns into colder wind, leaves turn dull and fall off the trees, and the days become noticeably short with gloomy skies. People suffer more pains in their body and joints. Emotions are in a state of "holding back" and people dislike being overly expressive in public. When winter comes, the weather reaches its most extreme state of cold. Everything freezes over, the earth cracks, water becomes ice, and people's emotions also stagnate. It can become easy to look at life in a more negative way, and negative thoughts may often come in dreams or suddenly appear in the mind.

Above all, late autumn and winter tend to have the most negative influence on people's emotions. In TCM, this is called yu (stasis), when emotions are easily caused by circumstances or environmental factors including cold and humidity. Those who smoke and drink heavily have constitutional phlegm that blocks energy channels, creating held energy (*qi yu*), which evolves into the blood (*xue yu*), and eventually suppresses the appetite (*shi yu*). In this cycle, pent up energy is held to the point of having physiological effects, and many times is just triggered by a change of weather. If people manage their yang levels, and regulate their energy and blood circulation, then they can avoid negative emotions that are due to the influence of the seasons.

In TCM, one day is also considered to be divided into four seasons: Early morning is spring, midday is summer, dusk is autumn and late night is winter. In the Yellow Emperor's book, this theory is used to explain some diseases and emotional disorders. Morning tends to be a lighter time of release and rising. Midday feels like a high point of peace with no problems, but at dusk complaints and negative emotions arise, and the worst time is at night.

Midnight is a point of deepest yin and midday, highest yang. In Chinese medicine, 2am is the turning point of yang energy: Disease can turn to death or recovery. If the energy is unable to turn, it means that yang cannot grow and overtake yin. At 4am, we find the quick rising time of yang energy; if it is unable to rise, this is also a pivotal moment.

In the early morning, yang energy rises like the sun, so a good breakfast encourages a healthy rise of yang energy. This is important because disorders and emotions are controlled by your physiological rise in energy. By midday, yang energy rises to its pinnacle. A relaxing good lunch maintains an orderly balance, and good energy—including carbohydrates, protein and warm foods—at lunch can purge toxins and ills from the body.

At dusk, the yang energy starts to dissipate and yin energy takes over. If dinner is too late, it can be difficult to support energy toward the end of the day. A weakened body is then more susceptible to illness, disease and emotional fluctuations. In the middle of the night, all our yang energy is hiding in the organs, a time of healing, and superficially, the body is weaker and more susceptible to outside factors and foreign elements. There is no energy to fight pathogenic elements, and disease can escalate to an unmanageable degree. Clinical research shows a greater number of people die at night.

It is important to mention that the season influences different emotions over a short, intermittent time (a few hours, a few days, a week) as opposed to the length of the entire season. Should one notice overly negative emotions, then they can be easily treated through stress-releasing methods or doing things that make you happy. These seasonal influences don't necessarily produce a seasonal-related disease. Only some people are susceptible to be influenced to an escalated degree in the autumn/winter seasons, perhaps those who may have worked indoors for years, who have weak constitutions, dislike exercise and tend to live in their heads more than their bodies, as well as those sensitive to cold. Depression, sympathetic nervous disorder or anxiety and fear are sometimes seen in these people. Medical research also has evidence that depression induced by the autumn or winter usually attacks people in adulthood, around the age of 23 and above. Females have four times the propensity to experience this.

For certain kinds of emotional disorders, combined with the physiological symptoms mentioned above and an inability to alleviate them through lifestyle changes, it is recommended the person seek a professional. Seasonal disorders can be quite serious, and the suicide rate is higher in countries where winter is particularly lengthy than in warmer areas. The group that is more easily influenced by seasonal depression needs more care during the winter, when symptoms tend to be more drastic. This is particularly the case if some life factor points are high, such as losing a family member.

In TCM, the late autumn season, when the atmosphere becomes drier, can easily affect the lung system. If dryness comes into the body, the lung system (nose, chest, surface of skin) is readily attacked by illness, causing lung yin deficiency. It is the lung system where sadness is stored in the body, so disruptions to this system can bring sadness or tearfulness, emotional ups-and-downs, excessive yawning or certain kinds of emotional irritability when things like one's career or relationship are not optimal. When disharmony between the liver and lung occurs, it disrupts the ascending and descending energy systems, and energy cannot be released properly. Bodily fluid metabolism is influenced: The throat feels choked, unable to disperse or clear phlegm.

In the winter season, the cold is a factor in pathogenic illnesses. Cold corresponds to kidney function. In TCM, the kidney is responsible for fear. Invasion of cold constricts the movement of energy and eventually damages the yang energy, causing a disharmony between the kidney yang and yin. The resulting stagnant blood circulation of the body and the kidney, the root of yin-yang for all the organs, can affect the overall balance of energy in the body. Some people will feel a blockage of energy and liquid from the lower abdomen up to the middle stomach and into the throat. This is called "counter-rising of qi and body fluids" and can be helped by regulating liver and kidney yang energy, which eventually will help water metabolism in the body.

The winter season may also play a part in a disorder of the autonomic nervous system. This system controls organs and puts them in the proper rhythm. The parasympathetic nervous system automatically takes over from the sympathetic nervous system in the evening, shutting down its "fight or flight" responses and allowing for a "rest and digest" response. If messages are sent at the wrong time, then after a while, your body and organs get confused about when to work and when to be active. Therefore, the *Yellow Emperor's Inner Canon* recommends going to sleep earlier in the autumn and winter seasons, exercising in the sunlight, and keeping calm and reserving emotions, so as to keep the system in balance.

Warming and tonifying kidney yang energy is one of the effective ways to regulate emotional disorders. Generally speaking, when autumn and winter come, we should take care of our yang energy as it goes into decline. When we experience more sadness or loneliness, or feel agitation from everyday life, we should counteract these feelings with light, exercise, music and creating an active environment to change the physiological and mental effects of the seasons on our body.

Remedy and Solution

Food options for treating symptoms of mild seasonal depression

Seasonal emotional changes vary according to the individual. Here we only provide advice for those who have emotional disturbance in autumn and winter. For seasonal winter depression, half an hour of outdoor exercise a day is recommended if it is sunny. Sunlight exercise is a more effective alternative therapy than traditional drugs for continuous and total recovery from seasonal depression.

Every day, our energy starts flowing when we have our breakfast. It is best to have a warm breakfast that has a good mix of various nutrients, like protein, good fat, fiber and carbohydrates.

Have functional food for breakfast, such as: Jujube 6 pieces, Chinese yam 15g, walnut 2 pieces, dolichos seed 扁豆 10g and edible pine nut 松子 10g.

Dry Chinese hawthorn berry 山楂 or carthamus flower 红花. Have 5g for tea.
(Good for cold and damp constitutions)

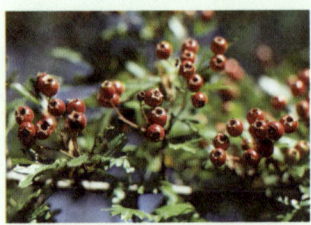
Hawthorn Berry

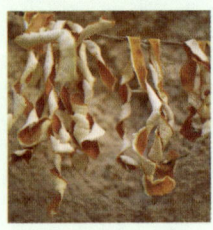
Tangerine Peel

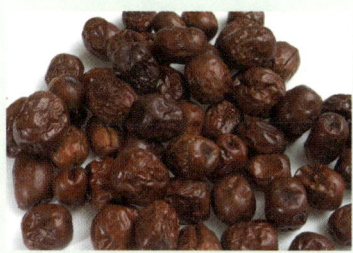
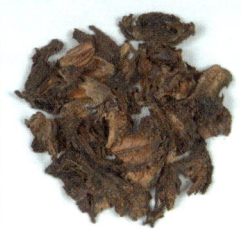

Small Jujube   Chaenomeles Lagenaria Koidz

Plum throat

Tangerine peel 陈皮 and Chinese rose flower 月季花. Use 5g of peel and 3 flowers for tea.
(Good for damp constitution)

Counter-rising of qi and body fluids

Cinnamon twig 桂枝 10g, white peony root 白芍 6g, fresh ginger root 生姜 6 pieces, licorice 甘草 4g, small jujube 小红枣 12 pieces. Add 1 liter of water, stew 30 minutes until there is 500ml of decoction. Divide into 2 portions and drink when it warm.
(Good for cold and weak constitutions)

Stiffness of neck and shoulder or calf spasm

Papaya 番木瓜 1 whole or Chaenomeles lagenaria Koidz 木瓜 10g. Steam with preserved rice wine for 30 minutes. Divide into two portions. Take one portion every night for 6 days.

Lingzhi Mushroom (*ling zhi* 灵芝)

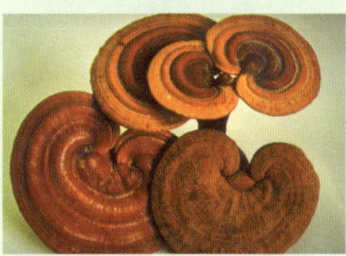

Lingzhi Mushroom
Photograph by Roy Upton, Courtesy of American Herbal Pharmacopoeia, Scotts Valley, CA

• **Therapeutic Taste and Property:** Bland, sweet or bitter depending on cultivar, neutral to warming.
• **Function:** Nourishes the heart and calms spirit-mind, relieves cough, tonifies qi and blood, supplements the kidney and stabilizes the will.
• **Application:** It is used to treat symptoms of heart and spleen deficiency manifesting as symptoms of insomnia, palpitations, forgetfulness, fatigue, listlessness and poor appetite.
• **Usage and Dosage:** 3-9g dry slices used in decoction or 1-1.5g of powdered extract for eating.

Self-Acupressure Point

The Diffusing Points (Shixuan 十宣)

Location: On the tips of the ten fingers, a few millimeters from the nail, in the center of the fingertips.
Function: Frees jaw and opens orifices. Reduces fever and settles pain.
Indication: Revive to consciousness, treat shock, fainting, epilepsy, coma, high-fever induced emotional hysteria, and infantile convulsions.

Method: Keep five fingers together on right, then make 30 circles on left in the center of the palm.

You can also massage the ear 5 times, then press with clockwise pressure 1/3 from the top of ear, 20 times each ear.

If you have complicated symptoms, please seek medical help to find out the reasons and have a thorough diagnosis.

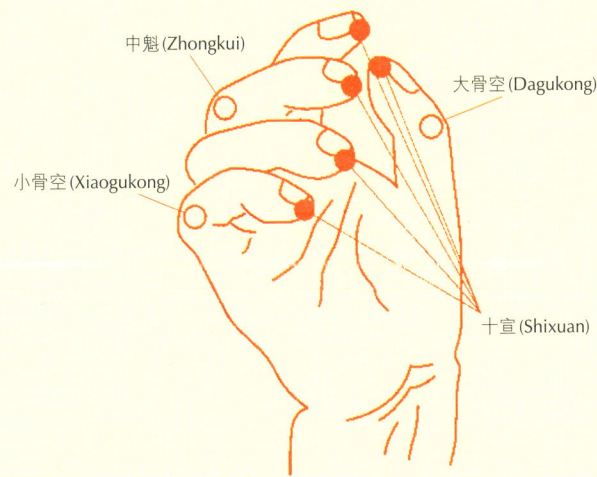

Appendices

Yin-Yang Theory

Principles and Formation

Yin and yang are the two fundamental principles or forces in the universe, ever opposing and supplementing each other. This ancient philosophical concept has become an important component of the basic theory of Traditional Chinese Medicine (TCM). There is no direct English translation of yin and yang, so the pinyin (a romanized expression of the sounds of the Chinese characters) is widely used.

In the beginning, yin and yang described a place's location in relation to the sun. A place exposed to the sun is yang, and a place without exposure is yin. The southern side of a mountain, for example, is yang, while its northern side is yin. Thus the ancient Chinese people, in the course of their everyday life and work, came to understand that all aspects of the natural world could be seen as having a dual aspect, for example, day and night, brightness and dimness, movement and stillness, upward and downward directions, heat and cold, etc.

The terms yin and yang are applied to express these dual and opposite qualities. Chapter Five of the ancient TCM classic *Book of Plain Questions* states that "water and fire are symbols of yin and yang" and that, furthermore, their interaction promotes the creation, development and transformation of things.

Yin-yang theory has had an integral impact on the science of TCM, and its basic principals have played an important role in the formation and development of TCM's own theoretical system.

The Content of Yin-Yang Theory

The content of the theory of yin and yang can be described briefly as follows: opposition, interdependence, relative waxing and waning, and transformation.

I) Opposition and Interdependence of Yin and Yang

By the opposition of yin and yang, we mean that all things and phenomena in the natural world contain two opposite components: heaven and earth, outside and inside, movement and stability, rising and falling, etc. In the theory of yin and yang, heaven is considered yang, while earth is yin; outside is yang, while inside is yin; movement is yang, while stability is yin.

Yin and yang not only oppose but also contain each other. Without the other neither can exist. For instance, there would be no earth without heaven, and vice versa. Without outside, there would be no inside, and vice versa. This relationship of coexistence is known as interdependence. TCM holds that "functional movement" belongs to yang, "nourishing substance" to yin, and that the one cannot exist without the other.

2) The Waxing and Waning of Yin and Yang and the Transformation between Yin and Yang

Yin and yang are not stagnant but exist in a dynamic

state—while yin wanes, yang waxes, and vice versa. This dynamic change of succeeding each other is known as the waxing and waning of yin and yang. Take the seasonal climatic variation in the natural world for example. The weather gets warm when winter gives way to spring, and becomes hot when spring gives way to summer, during which time yin wanes while yang waxes. However, it gets cool when autumn replaces summer, and cold when winter replaces autumn, during which time yang wanes but yin waxes.

By "transformation," we mean yin and yang will transform into one another under certain conditions. For instance, in the course of suffering from a disease, a patient may run a high fever, have a red complexion, feel irritable and restless, and have a rapid and strong pulse—indicating strong yang. But all of a sudden, he may show yin characteristics, feeling listless, with a low temperature, pale face and weak pulse. This is an example of transformation from yang to yin.

Uses of Yin-Yang Theory in TCM

Yin-yang theory is embodied in every aspect of TCM's theoretical system. It is used to explain the body's composition, its physiology functions and pathology changes, and to direct clinical diagnosis and treatment.

The yin-yang theory can also be used to summarize the property, flavor and function of foods and medicinal herbs, and this forms a basis for their clinical application. For example, food and herbs with a cold or cool nature belong to yin, while food and herbs with a warm or hot nature are yang. Food and herbs with sour, bitter and salty flavors belong to yin, while the food and herbs with pungent, sweet and bland to yang. In TCM, the principles of treatment are based on the predominance or weakness of yin and yang, so food and herbs are selected as remedies according to their specific properties. In doing so, one can achieve the aim of curing diseases.

Five Elements Theory

The Conception and Formation of Five Elements Theory

In Chinese, the Five Elements are called *Wu Xing*—*Wu* means five and *Xing* means movement and change. The Five Elements are: wood, fire, earth, metal and water. These elements each have their own special properties, which are at the root of the ancient philosophical concepts used in TCM.

Although the Chinese theory of Five Elements and the Greek theory of Four Elements are different in their history of formation, the rudiments of both belong to the earliest atomic theory. In order to explain the material world around them, ancient philosophers made a generalization and deduction about the respective properties of the substances and their interactive relationships. According to Chinese theory, wood, fire, earth, metal and water are the five basic substances that constitute the material world. They each have their own specific properties, but they also play interactive generation and restriction functions, and are in a constant state of motion and change.

The Content of the Theory of Five Elements

1) Classification in the Natural World

In light of Five Elements theory, TCM has made a comprehensive study of all things in nature, including the human body, and attributed them respectively to one of the Five Elements, in accordance with their different properties, functions and forms. Thus the theory shows the strong correlation between humans and their natural surroundings.

Classification According to Five Elements Theory

Human Body

Five Elements	Zang-Organs	Fu-Organs	Five Sense Organs	Five Tissues	Emotional Activity
Wood	Liver	Gall bladder	Eye	Tendon	Anger
Fire	Heart	Small Intestine	Tongue	Vessel	Joy
Earth	Spleen	Stomach	Mouth	Muscle	Thinking
Metal	Lung	Large Intestine	Nose	Skin and Body Hair	Worry
Water	Kidney	Urinary Bladder	Ear	Bone	Fear

Nature

Five Elements	Season	Environmental Factors	Growth & Development	Color	Taste	Orientation
Wood	Spring	Wind	Germination	Blue	Sour	East
Fire	Summer	Heat	Growth	Red	Bitter	South
Earth	Rainy Season	Dampness	Transforming	Yellow	Sweet	Middle
Metal	Autumn	Dryness	Reaping	White	Pungent	West
Water	Winter	Cold	Storing	Black	Salty	North

2) Relationships among the Five Elements

Among the Five Elements, there are relationships of generation, restriction, subjugation and reverse restriction.

Generation implies production and promotion. The order of generation is as follows: Wood generates fire, fire generates earth, earth generates metal, metal generates water, water generates wood.

The relationship of generation is composed of two aspects—generating and being generated. The element that generates is called the mother, while the element that is generated is called the son. Hence, the relation of generating and being generated is also known as that of mother and son. Take wood for example. Because wood produces fire, it is called the mother of fire. On the other hand, wood is produced by water, so it is called the son of water.

Restriction connotes bringing under control or restraint. In Five Elements theory, restriction works in the following order: Wood restricts earth, earth restricts water, water restricts fire, fire restricts metal, and metal restricts wood. Each can both restrict and be restricted. Take wood for example: Wood is restricted by metal, while wood, in turn, restricts earth.

In the interactive material world, neither generation nor restriction is dispensable. Without generation, there would be no birth and development; without restriction, excessive growth would result in harm. In generation, there resides restriction, and in restriction there exists generation.

The Five Elements oppose each other and at the same time cooperate with each other. When a relative balance is maintained between generation and restriction, normal growth and development is ensured. Should one of the Five Elements be excessive or insufficient, the phenomena of abnormal restrictions appear, known as subjugation (over-restriction) and reverse restriction. Generation and restriction are normal relationships among the Five Elements. Subjugation and reverse restriction are abnormal relationships of restriction.

Subjugation follows the order of restriction, and means that one element subdues the other when one becomes too strong or the latter is weak. It is the manifestation of abnormal coordination among things. For instance, if wood is in excess or earth is insufficient, and metal cannot exercise normal restriction on wood, then the excessive wood will subjugate earth, causing earth to become weaker.

Reverse restriction means preying upon others. It follows an order opposite to restriction. That is, when any one of the Five Elements is in excess, the one that originally restricts it will be restricted by it instead. That is why we call it reverse restriction. For instance, the normal order of restriction is that wood restricts earth; but if earth is in excess or wood is insufficient, earth will restrict wood in the reverse direction. It is clear that the order of reverse restriction is opposite, and is undoubtedly a harmful one.

The Application of Five Elements Theory in TCM

In the science of TCM, the theory of Five Elements is mostly used to explain the physiology functions of organs, and pathology changes of the human body and their relationship. Therefore, it guides clinical diagnosis and treatment. The Five Elements theory is often combined with yin-yang theory in TCM.

TCM Psychological Theory in Relation to the Five Elements

The generation and restriction relationship among the

Five Elements has a guiding significance in treating mental disorders. In the clinic, treatment applies the mutual restriction relationship between emotions in order to regulate them. For example, the *Yellow Emperor's Inner Canon* states:

"Over-anger impairs the liver, sadness/grief subdues anger."

"Over-joy impairs the heart, fear subdues joy." (See Chapter 2 for an example of over-happiness treated with fear.)

"Over-longing or pensiveness impairs the spleen, anger subdues longing or pensiveness." (See Chapter 3 for an example of over-longing treated with anger.)

"Over-worry impairs the lung, joy subdues worry."(See Chapter 3 for an example of over-worry treated with joy.)

"Over-fear impairs the kidney, but pensiveness subdues fear."

Five Systems of the Body

Our definition of the five organs includes both the organ and their functional system, which are linked via meridians and operate in conjunction with the entire body.

Heart system: heart—small intestine—blood vessels—tongue

Liver system: liver—gall bladder—tendons—eyes

Spleen system: spleen—stomach—muscles—mouth

Lung system: lung—large intestine—skin and body hair—nose

Kidney system: kidney—urinary bladder—bone—ears and lower orifices

Brief Patient Diagnosis

Patient diagnosis in TCM has many differences with the diagnosis procedures used in Western medicine. In TCM, this is the general process I go through to diagnose patients:

First, I look at the patient's physical build, facial complexion and eyes. Then, I observe standing and sitting posture, hear the quality of the patient's voice, and begin to talk and understand the logic and speed of responses in conversation. I look at the patient's eyes to determine the shine and shape, which relates to the organs. I examine the tongue to understand the state of the patient's qi and any invasion of factors as determined from tongue coating. Finally, I look under the tongue to see the flow of blood throughout the body.

Taking a person's pulse is a vital part of the examination. While in Western medicine, this only means counting heartbeats per minute, TCM undertakes a detailed evaluation of the heartbeat. I first take the *Cun Guan Chi* or Three Pulses to determine the "floating, medium and deep level" of meridian and organ energy flow. For instance, in a normal pulse, my three fingers can feel the strength of the pulse on the medium or middle level. If I can only feel the pulse on a deep level with one or two fingers, there is most likely a deficiency.

It is also important to detect the rhythm of the pulse, which indicates whether the flow is in the right rhythm, controlling the mood and "ups and downs" of the person. An even, steady beat equals an even, steady mood. Finally, I feel the flow of blood in the vessels, whether the quantity feels adequate and the stream of blood is strong.

Sometimes left and right hands both need to be felt for a more thorough analysis.

I will also look at a person's nails to assess the digestive system and how well the person assimilates vitamins and minerals. A white tip and cuticle with a flexible nail shows the health and vitality of a person. The color, texture and quality of the nails are also linked with the quality of one's liver blood.

Similarly, I look at a person's teeth, to understand the strength of the kidney system. If a calcium-deficient person takes a lot of calcium supplements, but has a weak kidney system, the person is still unlikely to absorb these supplements. For some people, I also look at skin color and texture, which is sometimes linked with the meridians as they control different portions of the skin.

Different Constitutions and Temperaments

(According to Original TCM Texts)

	Constitution	Temperament
Tai Yin	more yin, no yang; sticky blood; *wei qi* slow; yin and yang not harmonized; soft tendons, thicker skin	from the outside looks modest, but inside is suspicious; over-thinking; pessimistic; cowardly; likes to be alone, keeps distance from others; slightly conservative; doesn't like to be excited

	Constitution	Temperament
Shao Yin	more yin, less yang; small stomach, bigger large intestine; *fu*-organs not harmonized	cold; deep thinking; self-controlled; internalizes thoughts; plans ahead; doesn't brag; does not take action until time is right; easily jealous; soft and weak
Tai Yang	more yang, very little yin	proud; self-confident; subjective; aggressive, ambitious; bold, daring; opinionated, brave; believes only in own judgment; very irritable and easily angered; stubborn, resolute; easily talks back
Shao Yang	more yang, less yin; energy and blood circulating in harmony; yin deficient	social and approachable, flourishes in social settings; happy, open-minded, sometimes can have fast reactions and be optimistic; charming and frivolous; likes to smile and talk, but does not easily act; lots of friends and likes entertainment; no discipline or perseverance
Yin Yang Balanced	yin and yang in balance; blood and energy harmonized	relaxed, harmonized, easy-going; honorable, dignified; modest and self-effacing; happiness nor anger shown on face but self-content and self-satisfied; disregards the need for anything other than what already have; brave, unselfish, undisturbed; can handle changes in society, adaptable

Helpful Acupressure Points

The Diffusing Points (Shixuan 十宣)

Location: On the tips of the ten fingers, a few millimeters from the nail.

Indication: Revive to consciousness, treat shock, fainting, epilepsy, coma, high fever induced emotional hysteria, and infantile convulsions.

Hall of Impression (Yintang 印堂)

Location: Between the eyebrows, equidistant from each eyebrow.

Indication: Treat muddy-headedness, headache, insomnia, and infantile convulsions. Release pent-up tension or excess yang in order to calm the body.

Water Trough (Shuigou 水沟)

Location: In the crease above the upper lip, one third of the distance from the base of the nasal septum to the red skin of the upper lip on the midline.

Indication: Treat mental disorder, epilepsy, hysteria, infantile convulsions, coma, and stroke.

Great Mound (Daling 大陵)

Location: At the midpoint of the inner wrist crease, between the two major tendons of the wrist.

Indication: Treat cardiac pain and palpitations, mental disorders, epilepsy, stuffy chest, pain in the hypochondriac region, palpitation due to fright, mania and withdrawal, insomnia, irritability, bad breath, and stomach ache.

Union Valley (Hegu 合谷)

Location: The fleshy part between the thumb and forefinger,

pressing down with the thumb of the other hand and with forefinger on the opposite side.
Indication: Treat headaches, muddy-headedness, open the chest to resolve stagnated lung qi and harmonize with large intestine.

Spirit Gate (Shenmen 神门)

Location: Between the first and second wrist crease, in the depression on the little finger side of your inner arm.
Indication: Treat cardiac pain, irritability, palpitations, hysteria, amnesia, insomnia, mania and epilepsy. Also helps balance the heart and liver.

Wind Pool (Fengchi 风池)

Location: On the posterior aspect of the neck, below the occipital bone (base of skull), on the hairline in a depression on the outer area of the largest tendon (on both right and left sides).
Indication: Treat headache of the shaoyang meridian, vertigo, difficulty going to sleep, blurred vision, tinnitus, convulsions, epilepsy, fibroid disease, common cold (open nasal tracts), and good for stagnation around the neck area caused by emotional upset.

Hundred Convergences (Baihui 百会)

Location: At the top of skull, on the middle line of the head, at the crossing of the line that runs vertically intersecting the nose with the line that runs from ear to ear.
Indication: Treat headache of the Jueyin meridian, mental disorder of sinking yang, prolapse of internal organs, coma, vertigo, and aphasia.

Quiet Sleep (Anmian 安眠)

Location: At the middle point of the depression behind the ear, next to the earlobe and the Fengchi point.
Indication: Treat insomnia, irritability, migraine, palpitations, mental disorder, light and disturbed sleep.

Middle Stomach (Zhongwan 中脘)

Location: On the upper abdomen, on the middle line, two fingers below the chest bone, in the depression.
Indication: Treat stomach ache, abdominal distension, nausea, vomiting, acid regurgitation, diarrhea, jaundice, indigestion caused by stress, insomnia, and palpitations.

Moving Between (Xingjian 行间)

Location: On the dorsal aspect of the foot, on the web area between the first and second toe, right at the line coloration of light and darker skin.
Indication: Treat irregular menstruation, insomnia, epilepsy, convulsions, premenstrual tension, swelling and painful chest, distension of the abdominals, pain and fullness of the hypochodrium, swelling and pain of the eyes, dizziness and vertigo.

Chinese Food and Herbs

Properties

The characteristics of food and herbs can be described through Four Temperatures and Five Flavors (*si qi wu wei* 四气五味), and their different channels of entry.

The Four Temperatures are: warm, hot, cool and cold. In addition to the four temperatures, there is also neutral.

The Five Flavors are: sour, bitter, sweet, pungent and salty. In addition to the five flavors, there are also three sub-flavors: astringent, bland and neutral.

Features and Application

Plant name	Chinese name	Temperature (Sl=slightly)	Taste	Functions	Dosage	Way of eating
Adzuki bean	赤小豆	Sl cold	Sweet, sour	Induce diuresis to remove edema; eliminate jaundice; clear heat; detoxify and treat boils	10~30g	Porridge (use with caution with yin deficiency)
Aloe vera	芦荟	Cold	Bitter	Promote healthy bowels	1~2g	Powder, beverage, yogurt
Angelica root	当归	Warm	Sweet, pungent, bitter	Fortify and regulate blood circulation; regulate menstruation and stop pain; nourish dryness and activate bowels	3~10g	Decoction, put in wine (contraindicated for hot constitution and bleeding, use caution with dampness in digestive system and diarrhea)
Apple	苹果	Cool	Sweet	Promote production of body fluid; nourish the lung; relieve restlessness and summer heat; stimulate appetite; dispel effects of alcohol	100~150g (fresh)	Raw, juice, jam, dessert, soak in wine
Artemisia annua herb	青蒿	Cold	Bitter, sl. pungent	Clear heat and summer heat; dispel yin deficiency fever; cut off malaria	3~9g	Decoction (use with caution with weak constitution)
Asparagus	芦笋	Cold	Sweet	Expel heat; nourish bodily fluids; remove water retention; help urethra infection	30~60g (fresh)	Fried, steamed (use with caution with cold/weak digestive system)

137

Plant name	Chinese name	Temperature (Sl=slightly)	Taste	Functions	Dosage	Way of eating
Astragalus root	黄芪	Warm	Sweet	Tonify qi; lift yang; enhance immune system to protect exterior of body; arrest sweating; induce diuresis to remove edema	6~15g	Boiling, soup, decoction (contraindicated for infection, yin deficiency with excess yang)
Bamboo leaf	淡竹叶	Cold	Sweet, bland	Clear away heat to relieve restlessness; clear heart fire; promote diuresis	5~10g	Decoction (contraindicated for empty cold constitution)
Barley	大麦	Cool	Sweet	Disperse liver energy stagnation; treat unhappiness, poor appetite, chest and abdominal bloating	15~20g	Boiled, mix with other herbs
Barley sprout (or malt)	麦芽	Neutral	Sweet	Remove food stagnation; return breast milk	10~15g	Decoction, powder (use with caution if pregnant or breast-feeding)
Black bean	黑大豆	Neutral	Sweet	Regulate blood circulation; remove water retention; ease spasm; strengthen digestive system and kidney	9~30g	Bean milk, porridge, powder
Black fungus	黑木耳	Neutral	Sweet	Invigorate qi, nourish blood; moisten lung; stop cough and bleeding	3~10g	Fried, soup (use with caution for cold and weak large intestine, diarrhea)

Plant name	Chinese name	Temperature (Sl=slightly)	Taste	Functions	Dosage	Way of eating
Black sesame	黑芝麻	Neutral	Sweet	Tonify blood and yin	10~15g	Oil, raw, fried
Boat-fruited sterculia seed	胖大海	Cool	Sweet, bland	Moisten lung and smooth throat; clear away heat; regulate bowels	1~2 pieces	Tea, decoction (use with caution with cold/weak digestive system, diarrhea)
Cabbage	卷心菜	Neutral	Sweet, pungent	Expel heat	50~100g	Raw, fried, soup
Carrot	胡萝卜	Neutral	Sweet	Strengthen digestive system; remove food stagnation	50~100g	Raw, fried, juice, soup
Cassia seed	决明子	Sl. cold	Sweet, bitter	Clear liver fire to improve eyesight; moisten intestines to relax bowels	3~9g	Tea, decoction (use with caution with cold/weak digestive system, diarrhea)
Celery	芹菜	Cool	Bitter, sweet	Remove dampness and water; cool heat	100g	Raw, fried
Chaenomeles lagenaria Koidz	木瓜	Warm	Sour	Relax muscles and tendons; activate qi and blood in the channels; ease stomach; remove dampness	5~10g	Decoction, powder, put in wine
Chamomile	洋甘菊 黄春菊叶	Cool	Bitter, sweet	Promote qi movement in liver, spleen, lung and pericardium	2~3g	Tea
Chicken	鸡	Warm	Sweet	Warm midsection; strengthen qi; nourish essence and marrow	100g	Soup, meat (use with caution with acute, existing disease)

Plant name	Chinese name	Temperature (Sl=slightly)	Taste	Functions	Dosage	Way of eating
Chinese cabbage	黄芽菜	Neutral	Sweet	Open up and smooth stomach and intestines; nourish stomach; induce urine	50~100g (fresh)	Fried, soup
Chinese hawthorn berry	山楂	Warm	Sweet, sour	Promote blood circulation; resolve phlegm	3-6g	Boiled, dry
Chinese leek seed	韭菜子	Warm	Pungent, sweet	Strengthen liver and kidney, fortify yang and secure the essence	3~9g	Porridge, decoction (contraindicated for those with "empty-fire")
Chinese lettuce root	莴苣	Cool	Bitter, sweet	Induce urine; increase breast milk; remove heat; detoxify	30~60g	Fried (use with caution for digestive system weakness)
Chinese millet	秫米	Cool	Salty	Strengthen spleen; calm mind; treat poor appetite and light sleeping	15~20g	Boiled, mix with other herbs
Chinese raspberry	覆盆子	Sl. warm	Sweet, sour	Fortify liver and kidney; secure the essence and reduce frequent urination; shine eyes	5~10g	Decoction, powder, put in wine (contraindicated for "empty heat" and less urine)
Chinese rose flower	月季花	Warm	Sweet, sl. bitter	Promote blood circulation; regulate menstruation; detoxify; relieve swelling	9~15g (fresh) 3~6g (dry)	Tea, decoction, or exterior use
Chinese yam	山药	Neutral	Sweet	Tonify qi and yin of lung, spleen and kidney; treat over-thinking's diarrhea, seminal emission and fatigue	50g (fresh) 10~30g (dry)	Boiled, fried steam, powder

Plant name	Chinese name	Temperature (Sl=slightly)	Taste	Functions	Dosage	Way of eating
Chrysanthemum	菊花	Sl. cold	Sweet, bitter, pungent	Counteract heat; remove toxins	2~3g	Tea
Cinnamon and twig	肉桂 桂枝	Hot (twig: warm)	Pungent, sweet	Supplement fire; strengthen yang; expel cold; alleviate pain; warm channels to promote blood circulation Twig: expel cold in exterior	1~3g 0.5~1.5g (powder) 1.5~3g (twig)	Powder, decoction Twig: decoction (contraindicated for deficiency fire, excess heat, bleeding and pregnancy)
Citrus fruits	柑橘	Cool	Sweet, sour	Remove heat; promote production of body fluid; dispel effects of alcohol; induce urine	30~50g (fresh) 10~12g (dry)	Fresh raw, juice, dry for tea (contraindicated for cold/weak digestive system)
Clove	丁香	Warm	Pungent	Counteract cold; promote qi circulation	0.5~1.5g	Tea, fried, as flavoring
Corn and silk	玉米 玉米须	Neutral	Sweet, bland (silk)	Corn: promote appetite, induce urine. Silk: induce urine, expel liver heat, clear gall bladder	30~60g 10~15g	Boiled, powder, decoction
Cortex Albziae bark and flower	合欢皮 合欢花	Neutral	Sweet	Tranquilize mind and disperse stagnant qi; activate blood circulation; relieve swelling	6~9g (bark) 3~6g (flower)	Decoction
Dolichos seed	扁豆	Neutral	Sweet, bland	Strengthen digestive system; dissolve dampness; expel summer heat; stop diarrhea	6~9g	Fried, powder, boiled

Plant name	Chinese name	Temperature (Sl=slightly)	Taste	Functions	Dosage	Way of eating
Edible pine nut (or pine kernel)	松子	Warm	Sweet	Promote production of body fluid; arrest convulsion; moisten lung; lubricate intestinal tract	6~9g	Raw, fried, baked
Evergreen tea	苦丁茶	Cold	Sweet, bitter	Expel liver heat; improve eyesight	3~6g	Tea, decoction
Fennel	小茴香	Warm	Pungent	Expel cold to alleviate pain; regulate stomach qi	1.5~3g	Tea, flavoring, decoction, fried
Fresh ginger root	生姜	Warm	Pungent	Counteract cold	3~6g	Tea, raw, fried
Ganoderma (or Lingzhi mushroom)	灵芝	Neutral to warm	Sweet, bland, or bitter depending on cultivar	Nourish and calm spirit, relieve cough, tonify qi and blood; supplement the kidney; stabilize will	6g (dry), 1~1.5g (powdered extract)	Decoction, powder, extract
Garlic	大蒜	Warm	Pungent	Detoxify; remove pesticide	6~9g	Raw, fried
Gingko nut	白果	Neutral	Sweet, bitter, astringent	Restrain lung qi and soothe asthma; reduce leucorrhea; reduce urination	3~6g	Boiled, fried (contraindicated for bacterial/viral infections) (note: poisonous if eaten raw)
Glutinous rice	糯米	Warm	Sweet	Tonify digestive system and lung; warm stomach; hidroschesis	20~30g	Wine, porridge, cakes, dumpling
Grape	葡萄	Neutral	Sweet, sour	Invigorate qi and enrich blood; strengthen bones and tendons; induce urine	50~100g (fresh)	Dry, raw, juice, soak in wine

Appendices

Plant name	Chinese name	Temperature (Sl=slightly)	Taste	Functions	Dosage	Way of eating
Green bean (or Mung bean)	绿豆	Cold	Sweet	Clear away pathogenic heat and toxic materials; remove summer-heat and induce diuresis; cure restlessness and thirst caused by summer-heat, edema, diarrhea, dysentery, erysipelas, carbuncle and swelling; relieve drug's toxicity	15~30g	Porridge, powder (use with caution with cold/weak digestion and diarrhea)
Green tea	绿茶	Sl. cold	Sweet, bitter	Resolve phlegm; drain water retention	3~6g	Tea
Honey	蜂蜜	Neutral	Sweet	Invigorate digestive system; stop cough; moisten dryness; detoxify	10~15g	With warm water, as jam (use with caution with dampness and diarrhea)
Jasmine flower	茉莉花	Warm	Pungent, slightly sweet	Regulate energy; open stagnation; remove dampness; harmonize digestive system	3~6g	Tea, soup, dessert, external use
Job's tear (or Pearl barley)	薏苡仁	Sl. cold	Sweet, bland	Promote diuresis to resolve dampness and invigorate digestive system; clear away heat to drain pus; resist cancer; calm spasm	15~30g	Soup, powder
Jujube (or Chinese red date)	红枣	Neutral	Sweet	Tonify blood and qi; calm mind	3~6 pieces	Boiled, tea, raw

143

Plant name	Chinese name	Temperature (Sl=slightly)	Taste	Functions	Dosage	Way of eating
Licorice	甘草	Neutral	Sweet	Tonify qi	6~9g	Boiled, tea, raw
Lily bulb	百合	Sl. cold	Sweet	Nourish lung yin; good for stress, depression and women with menopause	6~9g	Boiled, fried
Longan fruit	龙眼	Sl warm	Sweet	Tonify qi and blood; promote blood circulation; reduce cold	3~6g	Fresh, steam, boiled, dry
Lotus seed, leaf and plumule	莲子 荷叶 莲心	Neutral	Sweet, astringent (leaf: bitter)	Preserve kidney essence; invigorate spleen and relieve diarrhea; nourish heart and tranquilize mind	10g (lotus seeds) 3~6g (dried leaf) 2g (plumule)	Dessert, fresh, decoction, soup, tea
Momordica Charantia L. (or Bitter melon)	苦瓜	Cold	Sweet, bitter	Clear heart and liver fire or heat; treat agitation and irritability	10~15g	Boiled, fried, make liquid for juice (use with caution if you often have stomach pain or acid taste in mouth)
Momordica fruit	罗汉果	Cool	Sweet	Clear lung heat; remove phlegm; stop cough; moisten bowels	9~15g	Tea, soup, decoction (use with caution with cold in lung and external cough)
Mutton	羊肉	Hot	Sweet	Warm midsection and kidney; strengthen qi	100g	Soup, meat (use caution with disease, heat condition)

Plant name	Chinese name	Temperature (Sl=slightly)	Taste	Functions	Dosage	Way of eating
Ophiopogon tuber	麦门冬	Sl. cold	Sweet, sl. bitter	Nourish lung yin; engender stomach liquid; expel heart fire; eliminate vexation	6~12g	Decoction, pills, internal or external use (contraindicated for those with deficiency of cold, diarrhea, phlegm cold cough)
Orange	橙子	Cool	Sour	Regulate qi; remove distention; dispel effects of alcohol	100~150g (fresh)	Raw, juice, dessert, jam
Oyster meat and shell	牡蛎肉 牡蛎壳	Cold	Sweet, salty	Nourish yin and blood; treat irritability and insomnia for people with hot constitution or in summer	120g (fresh) 30g (dry shell)	Fried, boiled
Papaya	番木瓜	Neutral	Sweet	Remove food stagnation; expel dampness; open channels	30~60g (fresh) 9~15g (dry)	Raw, steam
Peach kernel	桃仁	Neutral	Sweet, bitter	Promote blood circulation; remove blood stasis; moisten intestine; relax bowels	3~6g	Break nuts to small pieces, decoction (use with caution if pregnant)
Peanut and leaf	花生 花生叶	Neutral	Sweet	Moisten lung; regulate stomach; arrest bleeding; treat dry cough, regurgitation, beriberi and hypogalactia; treat bleeding diseases of the internal organs and hemophilia	5~10g	Boiled

Plant name	Chinese name	Temperature (Sl=slightly)	Taste	Functions	Dosage	Way of eating
Pearl powder	珍珠粉	Cold	Sweet, salty	Calm spirit, relieve fear; expel liver heat; brighten eyes; detoxify; engender muscles	0.3~1g	Powder, external and internal use (use with caution if pregnant)
Peony root	白芍	Sl. cold	Bitter, sour	Nourish blood; relieve spasm to stop pain; astringe yin; suppress hyperactive liver	3~6g	Decoction (use with caution with deficiency cold)
Pepper	辣椒	Hot	Pungent	Warm digestive system; expel cold; direct qi downward; remove food stagnation	1~3g	Flavoring, powder
Polygonum (or Foti root)	首乌	Sl. warm	Bitter, sweet, astringent	Nourish blood and yin; stimulate bowel movements; stop itchiness of skin; detoxify	5~10g	Decoction, jelly, jam, soak in wine, powder (use with caution with phlegm-dampness, avoid using ironware)
Pumpkin and seed	南瓜 南瓜子	Neutral	Sweet	Invigorate spleen and stomach; replenish qi; relieve inflammation and pains; induce diuresis to remove edema; remove toxic materials of any substance; destroy intestinal parasites	20~30g	Soup; seeds can be powdered

Plant name	Chinese name	Temperature (Sl=slightly)	Taste	Functions	Dosage	Way of eating
Radish	萝卜	Cool	Pungent, sweet	Remove food stagnation; expel phlegm and heat; direct qi downward; smooth digestive system; detoxify	50~100g	Raw, fried, soup, external use (contraindicated for cold/weak digestive system)
Radish seed	莱菔子	Neutral	Pungent, sweet	Remove food stagnation; expel phlegm; direct qi downward	3~6g	Decoction (use with caution with spleen qi weakness)
Radix Polygalae	远志	Sl. warm	Pungent, bitter	Tranquilize mind; eliminate phlegm for resuscitation; dissipate carbuncles	3~6g	Decoction
Schisandra berry	五味子	Warm	Sour, astringent	Calm mind; fortify qi and kidney; engender fluids, enhance immune system to protect body surface; clear empty toxic heat; relieve cough	2~5g 1~3g (powder)	Decoction, powder
Semen armeniacae amarum almond	苦杏仁	Sl. warm	Bitter	Relieve cough and dyspnea; moisten intestine and relax bowels	3~6g	Break nuts into small pieces, decoction (use caution with dosage in infants)
Semen biota seed	柏子仁	Neutral	Sweet	Nourish heart and tranquilize mind; moisten intestine and relax bowels	3~6g	Decoction

Plant name	Chinese name	Temperature (Sl=slightly)	Taste	Functions	Dosage	Way of eating
Semen Euryales	芡实	Neutral	Sweet, astringent	Stabilize will and calm spirit-mind; solidify kidney and astringent essence; firm spleen and stop diarrhea	15~20g	Decoction, powder
Semen Ziziphus spinosa	酸枣仁	Neutral	Sweet, sour	Nourish heart; tonify liver; tranquilize mind; stop excessive perspiration	6~12g (decoction) 1.5~3g (powder)	Decoction, powder
Soy bean	黄大豆	Neutral	Sweet	Strengthen digestive system; expel food stagnation; remove water retention	30~50g	Bean milk, powder
Straw mushroom	草菇	Cold	Sweet	Expel summer heat, resist cancer, increase life expectancy	30~50g (fresh) 9~15g (dry)	Fried, soup
Tangerine peel	陈皮	Warm	Pungent, bitter	Regulate qi; harmonize spleen and stomach; eliminate dampness; resolve phlegm	3~6g	Decoction (use with caution with qi and yin weakness)
Tiger lily buds	黄花菜 忘忧草 金针菜	Sl. cold	Sweet	Cool liver; ease depression and perturbed feelings	10~15g	Boiled and fried (note: poisonous if eaten fresh)
Turmeric rhizome	姜黄	Warm	Bitter, pungent	Remove blood stasis and regulate qi; induce menstruation and stop pain	3~6g	Decoction, powder (use with caution with deficiency of blood and pregnancy)

Plant name	Chinese name	Temperature (Sl=slightly)	Taste	Functions	Dosage	Way of eating
Walnut	核桃仁	Warm	Sweet	Tonify kidney to arrest spontaneous emission; warm lung to relieve asthma; moisten intestines to relax bowels	6~12g	Raw, powder
Wheat	小麦	Sl. cold	Sweet	Tonify heart and spleen; remove heat and agitation	15~30g	Soup, steam, bread
White fungus (or Silver ear)	银耳	Neutral	Sweet, bland	Nourish yin and engender fluids; moisten lung and stomach	3~10g	Dessert, soup (contraindicated for those with flu/cold and productive cough)
Wolfberry	枸杞子	Neutral	Sweet	Nourish yin; increase blood and essence; brighten eyes	6~9g	Fresh, steam, boiled, tea, raw, fried

All nations have their own traditional wisdom for living healthy. Let's share it! Then there will be much more knowledge for all ...

Bibliography

English:

1. Zhang Enqin, and Shi Lanhua etc. *Basic Theory of Traditional Chinese Medicine (I and II)*. Shanghai: Publishing House of Shanghai College of Traditional Chinese Medicine, 1989, 1990.
2. Zuo Yanfu, and Tang Decai. *Science of Chinese Materia Medica*. Shanghai: Publishing House of Shanghai University of Traditional Chinese Medicine, 2003.
3. Cheng Xinnong. *Chinese Acupuncture and Moxibustion*. Beijing: Foreign Languages Press, 1987.
4. Nigel Wiseman, and Andrew Ellis. *Fundamentals of Chinese Medicine*. Revised edition. US: Paradigm Publications, 1996.
5. Zhang Enqin, and Zhang Wengao etc. *Chinese Medicated Diet*. Shanghai: Publishing House of Shanghai College of Traditional Chinese Medicine, 1990.
6. Zuo Yanfu, and Wu Changguo. *Basic Theory of Traditional Chinese Medicine*. Shanghai: Publishing House of Shanghai University of Traditional Chinese Medicine, 2002.
7. Beijing University of Traditional Chinese Medicine. *Basic Theories of Traditional Chinese Medicine*. Beijing: Academy Press [Xue Yuan], 1998.
8. Zhang Qian. *The Change of Life—An End of a Woman's Reproductive Years*. Shanghai Daily, 02 February, 2008, p. C2.
9. Library of Chinese Classics. *Yellow Emperor's Canon of Medicine, Plain Conversation*. Chinese-English. Beijing, Shanghai, Guangzhou, Xi'an: World Publishing Corporation, 2005.
10. Giovanni Maciocia. *The Foundations of Chinese Medicine*. London: Churchill Livingstone, 1989.

Chinese:

1. 张继泽等:《张泽生医案医话集》,江苏科技出版社,1981年。
2. 张艳芳主编:《中医藏象学》,中国协和医科大学出版社,2004年。
3. (美)戈尔曼·丹尼尔:《情感智商》,上海科学技术出版社,1997年。
4. 匡调元:《人体体质学——理论应用和发展》,上海中医学院出版社,1991年。
5. 何裕民等:《中医性别差异病理学》,上海科学普及出版社,1997年。
6. 何裕民:《中国传统精神病理学》,上海科学普及出版社,1995年。
7. 刘增垣等:《心身医学》,上海科技教育出版社,2000年。
8. 黄跃东:《中医临床治疗精神疾病》,上海科学技术出版社,1998年。
9. 窦国祥:《饮食治疗指南》,江苏科学技术出版社,1981年。
10. 程士德主编,王洪图、鲁兆麟编:《素问注释汇粹》,人民卫生出版社,1982年。
11. 南京中医学院中医系:《黄帝内经灵枢译释》,上海科学技术出版社,1986年。
12. 南京中医药大学:《中药大辞典》,上海科学技术出版社,2006年。
13. 王效道等:《〈内经〉心理思想研究》,内部资料,1984。

```
RA          Yifang, Zhang,
790.53      1959-
.Y54
2009        Managing your
              emotional health
              using traditional

                       35019000029636
```

DATE			

South University Library
Richmond Campus
2151 Old Brick Road
Glen Allen, Va 23060

BAKER & TAYLOR